VARICOSE VEINS: SYMPTOMS, CAUSES AND TREATMENTS

PUBLIC HEALTH
IN THE 21ST CENTURY

NEUROANATOMY RESEARCH
AT THE LEADING EDGE

PUBLIC HEALTH IN THE 21ST CENTURY

VARICOSE VEINS: SYMPTOMS, CAUSES AND TREATMENTS

ANDREA L. NELSON
EDITOR

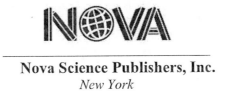

Nova Science Publishers, Inc.
New York

For permission to use material from this book please contact us:
Telephone 631-231-7269; Fax 631-231-8175
Web Site: http://www.novapublishers.com

NOTICE TO THE READER
The Publisher has taken reasonable care in the preparation of this book, but makes no expressed or implied warranty of any kind and assumes no responsibility for any errors or omissions. No liability is assumed for incidental or consequential damages in connection with or arising out of information contained in this book. The Publisher shall not be liable for any special, consequential, or exemplary damages resulting, in whole or in part, from the readers' use of, or reliance upon, this material. Any parts of this book based on government reports are so indicated and copyright is claimed for those parts to the extent applicable to compilations of such works.

Independent verification should be sought for any data, advice or recommendations contained in this book. In addition, no responsibility is assumed by the publisher for any injury and/or damage to persons or property arising from any methods, products, instructions, ideas or otherwise contained in this publication.

This publication is designed to provide accurate and authoritative information with regard to the subject matter covered herein. It is sold with the clear understanding that the Publisher is not engaged in rendering legal or any other professional services. If legal or any other expert assistance is required, the services of a competent person should be sought. FROM A DECLARATION OF PARTICIPANTS JOINTLY ADOPTED BY A COMMITTEE OF THE AMERICAN BAR ASSOCIATION AND A COMMITTEE OF PUBLISHERS.

Additional color graphics may be available in the e-book version of this book.

Library of Congress Cataloging-in-Publication Data

Varicose veins : symptoms, causes, and treatments / editor, Andrea L. Nelson.
       p. ; cm.
   Includes bibliographical references and index.
   ISBN 978-1-61209-841-8 (hardcover : alk. paper)
   1. Varicose veins. I. Nelson, Andrea L.
   [DNLM: 1. Varicose Veins. WG 620]
   RC695.V34 2011
   616.1'43--dc22
                                                                    2011004968

Published by Nova Science Publishers, Inc, + New York

CONTENTS

PREFACE

When veins become varicose, the leaflets of the valves no longer meet properly, and the valves do not work. This allows blood to flow backwards and they enlarge even more. Varicose veins are most common in the superficial veins of the legs, which are subject to high pressure when standing. This new book presents topical research in the study of the symptoms, causes and treatments of varicose veins. Topics discussed include segmental failure of the vaso-regulatory function of venous microcirculation causing varicose veins; the role of inflammation in varicose vein pathology; treatment of varicose veins by ultrasound-guided foam sclerotherapy and diagnostic airplethysmography.

Chapter 1 - The chapter defends the proposal that segmental failures of a vaso-regulatory function of the venous microcirculation, by increasing the dilator effect that plasma norepinephrine (NE) in the microcirculation has on veins, are the cause of varicose veins. Because the concepts of the microcirculation having a significant regulatory role, as distinct from a nutritional, and of circulating plasma NE having a hormonal venodilator potential are not generally recognized, the first three sections of this five section chapter are devoted to describing the circumstances and evidence from which the concepts have evolved and, then, in demonstrating how the concepts have been manipulated experimentally to create acute varicosities on a perfused segment of the canine lateral saphenous vein. The fourth section of the chapter demonstrates that the findings in acute experimental varicosities match, in detail, those found in pathological varicosities or else they provide a ready explanation of how they probably arise. The final section of the chapter offers a possible rationale for NE having two concurrent opposing effects in the cardiovascular system that is based on the chemosensory nature of smooth muscle and the evidence that all primary stimuli exhibit excitor and lateral inhibitory effects.

Chapter 2 - The pathogenesis of chronic venous disease, a complex and common pathology affecting the lower extremities, is still poorly understood. Accumulating evidence supports the role of inflammation as a mechanism underlying the physiopathology of chronic venous disease. In this review, we will carry out an overview of the role of inflammation in the varicose vein pathology, focusing on recent data that supports the use of pharmacological tools to decrease the production of inflammatory mediators or to block their effects, as a complementary therapeutic approach.

The most accepted mechanism linking venous hypertension to the changes in the macro and microcirculation is the leukocyte "trapping" model, according to which leukocytes infiltrate the venous wall and valves and migrate across the postcapillarvenules endothelium, thus leading to wall remodeling and valvular destruction. An incipient inflammatory focus in the vascular intima or media, the activation of endothelial cells by hypoxia, or altered hemodynamics, might cause the leukocytes to leave the circulation. In addition, fluid shear stress can contribute to leukocyte activation, and nitric oxide donors and inflammatory mediators can modulate the response. In the last decade, several reports have shown the involvement of molecules implicated in the inflammatory response such as adhesion molecules and cytokines, especially vascular cellular adhesion molecule-1, transforming growth factor-β, interleukin (IL)-6, IL-8 and matrix metalloproteinases, as well as the transcription factor hypoxia inducible factor-1 α in varicose vein disease. Additionally, in support of the leukocyte "trapping" model, recent data from our group has disclosed a correlation between elevated levels of chemotactic cytokines and varicose veins, specifically monocyte-chemo attractant protein-1, IL-8, interferon-inducible protein-10, RANTES, macrophage-inflammatory protein (MIP)-1α and MIP-1β. Furthermore, recent findings show that acetylsalicylic acid (ASA) treatment of patients with varicose syndrome accelerated healing and delayed recurrence of venous ulceration, suggesting that drugs that diminish leukocyte activation seemed to benefit ulcer healing and could be used as a complementary treatment. In addition to studies with human tissues, several animal model studies have suggested that inhibition of the early stages of inflammation offers potential targets that could be effective for the treatment of venous disease. In summary, recent reports highlight the impact of inflammation and hypoxia on varicose vein pathogenesis, and open the avenue to future preventive and therapeutic designs.

Chapter 3 - Partially due to the lack and difficulty in conducting longitudinal studies on the natural history of primary varicose veins, the pathophysiologic mechanisms that lead to the development and progression of vein reflux in lower limbs is unknown. Increasing evidence suggests that the development of primary venous insufficiency can follow an ascending pattern where the terminal valve is the last to be involved. This is conflicting with the traditional "retrograde" theory stating that the incompetence of valves above the saphenofemoral junction is the primary source of varicose disease that proceeds in a retrograde manner with progressive dilatation and valvular incompetence along the saphenous vein (SV) and its tributaries.

The ascending evolution is supported by hemodynamic principles, literature data and direct observations.

According to scientific laws, the development of venous insufficiency in lower limb is likely determined by the hydrostatic column of venous pressure and thereby follows the gravity gradient along the column. The lower the level (higher the gravity force), the higher the hydrostatic pressure causing venous incompetence and the reflux to begin. Once started a lower point, varicose vein disease can subsequently evolve uprising in accordance with the pressure gradient.

There is evidence to support that terminal valve involvement in varicose disease of SV can occur in less half population with SV insufficiency . In 45-55% of cases refluxes along SV are found below competent terminal valves that are therefore last components of SV to be involved from venous insufficiency.

Studies using selective and minimally invasive approach to treat varicose veins have also shown that after treatment localized in a target vein, the shrinkage and recovery of the of dilated varicose vein above can occur. This could not be explained with a retrograde development of varicose disease where the disease at above levels was antecedent and prelude to the involvement of lower venous segments.

The natural history of varicose veins is that of a progressive disease which chronic evolution. Although the exact development is uncertain, it is likely that the disease begins at the lower levels of the limbs and develops in an antegrade manner as venous stasis is higher where force of gravity is higher. This data do not support an aggressive and widespread treatment of the saphenous terminal valve as first strategy in the presence of varicose veins of lower limbs.

Chapter 4 - After the introduction of foam form of sclerosing solution, foam sclerotherapy rapidly gained its popularity. Nowadays, variety of venous disorder can be treated with foam sclerotherapy with low rate of adverse events. This Chapter presents the efficacy and safety of ultrasound-guided foam sclerotherapy for varicose veins and updates previous publications.

Chapter 5 - The objectives of the examination of venous abnormalities are to determine whether the problem is the result of outflow obstruction, reflux, or both, and to define the anatomic location; in addition, quantitative hemodynamic information is generally collected. Duplex ultrasonography is a useful test for the evaluation of reflux and obstruction of individual veins; however, it provides little quantitative hemodynamic information.

The ambulatory venous pressure (AVP) is the gold standard for functional and quantitative testing of the venous system of the lower extremities. The AVP is obtained by placing a catheter into a superficial vein of the lower leg. Pressure changes are recorded while the patient exercises the calf muscle pump by walking, rising up on tiptoes, or performing ankle dorsiflexion movement. Direct measurement of the AVP is the most reliable way to evaluate venous function; however, it is rarely used in clinical practice because of its invasive and time-consuming requirements. Instead, various plethysmography (air, strain gauge, impedance, photo) techniques have been developed for clinical use with the aim of replacing AVP measurements; plethysmograpic techniques quantitate the degree of reflux, obstruction, and/or calf muscle dysfunction by measuring changes in calf volume on various maneuvers.

Strain plethysmography measures the electrical resistance and is plotted on a strip chart, using a mercury strain gauge placed around the extremity. Change in volume causes a change in circumference and therefore in the length and electrical resistance of the strain. Impedance plethysmography measures the electrical impedance, which is inversely proportional to the volume. Photo plethysmography measures the reflection of infrared light by red blood cells in the cutaneous capillaries. Dorsal or plantar flexion of the foot reduces the amount of blood in the dermal plexus. On cessation of exercise, photoplethysmography records the capillary refilling time related to the dermal circulation. Airplethysmography (APG) is a technique used for measuring the pressure or volume changes in the lower limb using an air chamber placed around the lower leg.

Chapter 6 – Despite primary venous insufficiency is one of the most common diseases, pathophysiology leading to varicose vein development is today not well understood and object of multiple conjectures. Unfortunately, due to the complexity in investigating a dynamic phenomenon with multiple evolutions, dissimilar populations and incomparable settings, large longitudinal studies on the natural history of varicose veins are lacking and the mechanisms behind the development and progression of reflux in primary superficial venous insufficiency still remain largely uncertain.

Over the years, diverging theoretical models based on multiple assumptions have been developed to explain the relationship between venous reflux and venous disease, one of the most debated issues being whether development of varicose veins occurs downward or upraises along the leg. This understanding has indeed relevant implications for treatment, since the initial ("starting") points of venous disease are usually the most severe compromised necessitating of more aggressive and earlier treatment. At the opposite, the last involved venous sites might not require any direct action since the disease can spontaneously reverse once the treatment is applied to the first and more severe involved points. Therefore, dissimilar theoretical models on varicose vein progression have provided opposite basis for the development of new and improvement of existing therapies. Today large open debate in the varicose vein pathophysiology field, where traditional and modern concepts oppose, still remains. Critical analysis of evidence is essential to support scientific progress and objectively understand which and on what extent each theory might be reliable.

Chapter 7 - Varicose veins (VVs) are commonly attributed to valvular incompetence resulting in reflux and retrograde venous dilatation. The occurrence of VVs in the absence of sapheno-femoral (SF), sapheno–popliteal (SP) or perforator incompetence (IC), and alterations in the collagen and elastin content of the extracellular matrix (ECM) has lead investigators to postulate that other, as yet poorly defined local and systemic factors may act individually or in concert to alter the structural integrity and function of the venous wall. The clinical and histological manifestations of VVs occur as a result of the disruption of the normal venous architecture due to remodeling of the ECM. Persistence of these systemic and local factors may predispose to the high rates of residual and recurrent varicosities seen after treatment. Although a number of growth factors, proteases and their inhibitors known to modulate the ECM have been implicated in the pathogenesis of VVs, their etiology remains unknown. The identification of potential candidate genes and specific cell markers expressed in response physiologic or pharmacologic stimuli and hemodynamic forces may provide additional insights into the factors that regulate remodeling of the ECM` and ultimately to the development of VVs.

In: Varicose Veins   ISBN 978-1-61209-841-8
Editor: Andrea L. Nelson   ©2011 Nova Science Publishers, Inc.

Chapter 1

VARICOSE VEINS ARE CAUSED BY SEGMENTAL FAILURES OF THE VASOREGULATORY ROLE OF THE VENOUS MICROCIRCULATION, MEDIATED BY PLASMA NOREPINEPHRINE

Thomas P Crotty[*]
University College Cork Medical and Health School, Cork, Ireland

ABSTRACT

The chapter defends the proposal that segmental failures of a vaso-regulatory function of the venous microcirculation, by increasing the dilator effect that plasma norepinephrine (NE) in the microcirculation has on veins, are the cause of varicose veins. Because the concepts of the microcirculation having a significant regulatory role, as distinct from a nutritional, and of circulating plasma NE having a hormonal venodilator potential are not generally recognized, the first three sections of this five section chapter are devoted to describing the circumstances and evidence from which the concepts have evolved and, then, in demonstrating how the concepts have been manipulated experimentally to create acute

[*] Thomas P Crotty, BA, LPh, MB, MSc, Department of Physiology, The Western Gateway Building, University College Cork Medical and Health School, Western Road, Cork, Ireland, Email address:drtpcrotty 1966@gmail.com, Phone: +353 (0)21 4205866/5867, Fax: +353 (0)21 4205370

varicosities on a perfused segment of the canine lateral saphenous vein. The fourth section of the chapter demonstrates that the findings in acute experimental varicosities match, in detail, those found in pathological varicosities or else they provide a ready explanation of how they probably arise. The final section of the chapter offers a possible rationale for NE having two concurrent opposing effects in the cardiovascular system that is based on the chemosensory nature of smooth muscle and the evidence that all primary stimuli exhibit excitor and lateral inhibitory effects.

SECTION 1.

Introduction

[Please note: unless otherwise stated, references to "reflux" refer to radial reflux, where flow from the vein lumen perfuses its own local microcirculation by radial retrograde flow. By contrast, reflux associated with incompetent valves is axial reflux.]

The focus of this five section chapter is to explain and defend the proposition that varicose veins are caused by segmental failures of a vaso-regulatory function of the venous microcirculation (the vasa venarum network) that result in segmental increases in the dilator effect that circulating plasma norepinephrine (NE) has on segments of normal veins, when the drug stimulates them through their adventitial surface. This hypothesis has evolved from an original observation that isoprenaline (ISO) constricted a short segment of the canine lateral saphenous vein when it was injected into its lumen through one of its major tributaries [1]. That observation naturally suggested plasma NE might, under similar circumstances, dilate rather than constrict a short segment of a vein, thereby causing a varicosity on it. I believe enough experimental data now exists to give that suggestion a strong credibility.

Because the concepts of the microcirculation having a regulatory function in relation to the macrocirculation and of resting concentrations of circulating plasma NE having a hormonal venodilator effect are novel and not accepted at present, the first three sections of this chapter are devoted to describing the circumstances and evidence from which those concepts have evolved. The first section of the chapter gives a brief summary of what led to the serendipitous observation that, in the final analysis, has been responsible for the concepts. The second section introduces the concept of the modular construction of the microcirculation and the macrocirculation. It describes how the modules function independently, though normally in concert, how they are perfused and drained, and how, in addition to factors like viscosity and pressure gradients, physiological turbulence and the vascular endothelium are important regulators of the volume of blood perfusing the modules. The second section describes the evidence of the venodilator potency of microcirculatory plasma NE and comments briefly on the unique pharmacology of the microcirculation. The third section deals first with the structure and the function of the valve agger, a little known structure that regulates the drainage and reflux perfusion of every module and whose physical failure is believed to be the final common trigger of the varicose vein cascade. The section then goes on to demonstrate how knowledge of the agger and of the dilator potency of microcirculatory NE have been manipulated to create acute experimental varicosities, using NE, or equally well, ACh, for the purpose. The fourth section seeks to validate the hypothesis under consideration by showing that the changes found in experimental varicosities either match those found in pathological varicosities, in detail, or else they provide a straight forward, unforced explanation of how they might arise. The fifth and final section of this chapter discusses the apparently wasteful conflict represented by the NE stimulus having two components with opposing cardiovascular effects. It proposes that the conflict can be explained by the fact that vascular smooth muscle is a biological chemosensor and, as such, its stimulus, like all primary biological stimuli investigated to date, necessarily contains two components that cause opposing effects and are commonly referred to as excitor and lateral inhibitory.

It is understandable why those with an interest in varicose veins would be skeptical of the hypothesis put forward here. Apart from the fact that no one has independently verified the experimental data on which it is based, the hypothesis involves concepts that are not currently recognized or accepted and, moreover, that run counter to a number of long established beliefs, such as, that the role of the microcirculation is nutritional and not regulatory, that plasma NE has no significant hormonal effect, either dilator or constrictor, at normal concentrations [2], and that the biological importance of endogenous NE lies virtually solely in its role as the principle transmitter of the sympathetic nervous system [2]. The hypothesis also questions the centuries old belief that the venous microcirculation of a healthy vein cannot be perfused by direct radial reflux from the vein's lumen. Consistent with that belief, every perfusion study of the venous microcirculation over the centuries has, without exception, involved orthograde perfusion of the network. For all those reasons, then, it is easy to understand why the present consensus is that factors intrinsic to the vein itself are responsible for varicose veins, among them incompetent valves, non-specific wall weakness, sustained high hemostatic pressure, racial and gender characteristics, etc.

However I have demonstrated that the microcirculation of a normal vein can be perfused by radial reflux, at physiological pressures [3]. I made the demonstration by first opening the tightly closed reflux channels of a perfused segment of the canine lateral saphenous vein by stimulating it with $3\mu M$ NE. I then introduced radial components into the axial velocity vector of the segment's perfusate by making its flow turbulent. Those components, by their radial dissipative effect, literally pumped perfusate from the lumen of the segment into its microcirculation through the open reflux channels, at a pressure of around 100 mmHg. Recently Driefaldt and his colleagues confirmed that radial reflux was possible *in vivo* in a healthy vein by publishing a video clip showing blood pulsing through the microcirculation of a venous graft when the clamps were removed after a coronary bypass procedure was completed [4].

It may be objected that a canine vein segment is not suitable for investigating varicose veins because dogs, like all quadrupeds, never develop the condition spontaneously. However, two proven animal models of the condition exist, rats [5] and dogs [6]. In both models, surgically induced A/V fistulas have, as they do in humans, caused varicosities that on investigation have been found to have the same histological features as those found in the human condition.

The observation that first suggested a pathological varicosity might be caused by a regulatory failure of a segment of the venous microcirculation was made during an investigation into the pharmacology of the canine lateral saphenous vein that I was engaged in as part of a post graduate degree course in Physiology. I had taken the course in the hope of securing an appointment to a pre-clinical teaching post in my *alma mater,* the Cork University Medical School, after working as an internist in West Hartford, Connecticut, for several years. I made the critical observation when I injected a homeopathically inspired low concentration of isoproterenol (ISO) into the plantar tributary of a perfused *in vitro* segment of the canine vein and found that, contrary to normal expectation, it constricted the segment. The injection was recognized as being highly speculative and was only made to satisfy a curiosity inspired by reading an intriguing article on Fluidic control systems in LIFE magazine [7]. NASA was developing those systems at a time when reliable computer chips had not yet become available to guide rockets in the hostile environment of outer space. The systems consisted of complex arrays of tubing and valves that relied on the effect of rebalancing the fluid distribution within the arrays, caused by deviations from the planned flight path of rockets, to generate signals to correct the deviations. I injected ISO into the tributary because I perceived a very tenuous similarity between the fluidic arrays and the vascular circulation and, on that basis, conjectured the complex hemodynamic events that occur at a tributary junction might possess latent fluidic properties that, together with the questionable potential of a homeopathically inspired low dose of ISO, would change the normal intralumenal effect of ISO from dilator to constrictor. Against expectations, that indeed is what appeared to happen when I injected a 3ml bolus of 1ng/ml ISO solution into the canine vein through its plantar tributary and caused the vein to constrict.

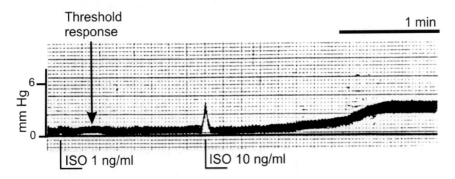

Figure 1. Recording showing a threshold response of the canine vein segment to isoproterenol 1ng/ml.

However, it soon became apparent that the constrictor effect was not caused by ISO having changed its intralumenal dilator effect into a constrictor effect. That conclusion was based on the fact that ISO had constricted the segment *upstream* of the junction of the injected tributary and *upstream* of a competent valve located between the site of constriction and the tributary junction [1]. Moreover the constrictor effect was confined to a short section of the segment, meaning ISO had created an acute stenosis of the segment at a concentration threshold about 45 times lower than that at which intralumenal NE was known to constrict the segment. Considered together, all the findings mentioned ruled out the possibility that ISO had constricted the segment by acting intralumenally. The problem then was to explain how it had acted. I finally had to accept what was, at the time, a highly unorthodox suggestion of my supervisor that the drug might have stimulated the segment through its microcirculation. While it subsequently proved easy to duplicate the stenotic effect consistently and to show it was dose dependent [1] it proved extremely difficult to prove that ISO had acted via the microcirculation by showing it was possible to stain the microcirculation at the site of the stenosis with ink injected along with ISO into the plantar tributary. That required more than a hundred injections, made over a number of years before, using a skin flap *in situ* preparation of the segment, I finally succeeded, for the first and only time, in staining a 5mm section of a single vas of the segment's microcirculation at the site of a stenosis (Fig2).

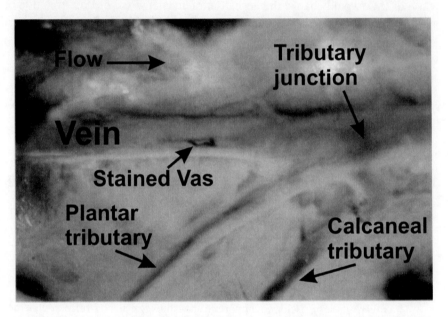

Figure 2. Photograph of an *in situ* skin preparation of the canine vein segment showing a single ink stained vas of the venous microcirculation, located upstream of the junction of the ink filled plantar tributary.

It took some time before I was able to establish that the vessel that had been responsible for transporting ISO to the site of the stenotic constriction from the tributary originated at the base of the cardinal valve of the tributary, located immediately distal to the tributary's junction (Fig.5).

At about the same time as I found ISO could constrict the canine segment I found NE could dilate it. The evidence of that was provided by the bimodal response patterns that the segment occasionally displayed when it had been stimulated by NE, either added to the perfusate or released by stimulating the segment electrically.

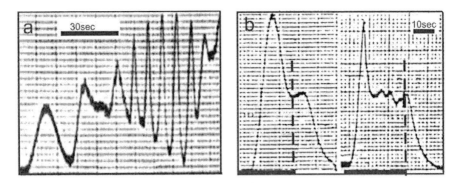

Figure 3. Records of bimodal responses of *in vitro* vein segments to (a) intralumenal NE and (b) electrical stimulation.

Because ISO was believed to have constricted the vein segment by stimulating it through its microcirculation it was reasonable to assume NE had dilated it in the same way. And because the effect of ISO had been limited to a short section of the segment it was reasonable to suppose the dilator effect of NE was similarly limited, meaning it had created a varicosity. Given my vicarious interest in varicose veins, kindled by an enthusiastic vascular surgeon during my intern days in St Mary's hospital in Waterbury, Connecticut, the possibility that varicose veins might be caused by plasma NE released from the microcirculation encouraged me to continue my research on the canine vein after I had been appointed to the staff of the medical school. Fortunately, my appointment was as a lecturer in Histology since that provided me with the special facilities I needed to be able to investigate the structural details of the reflux pathway I believed was involved in the microcirculatory effects of ISO and NE. Thanks to the courtesy of a succession of heads of the Physiology Department over the years, I was able to continue my investigation of the functional aspects of the canine segment.

SECTION 2.

The Experimental Design

A constant flow perfusion technique was used to investigate the responses of 5-10cm long, doubly cannulated segments of the canine lateral saphenous vein to drugs and electrical stimulation. Initially *in vitro* segments were used in the investigation [8] and later *in situ* segments, sited in hindlimbs that had been amputated at the knee joint [9]. Segments were perfused with oxygenated Tyrode solution at 34°C, at flow rates ranging between 32-38 ml /min, depending on segment diameters. Drugs were normally added to the perfusion reservoir. Directly recorded pressure changes in the perfusion circuit were used to determine if a segment was constricting or dilating - a rise in pressure indicated it was constricting, a fall that it was dilating. When a photograph of the physical change associated with a segment's response was required the perfusion pump was switched off at the appropriate stage of the response and a pH 6.6-6.8 solution of 2% glutaraldehyde and 2.5% paraformaldehyde in phosphate buffer was injected rapidly into the lumen of the segment, though a three way tap.

In vitro segments were stimulated electrically through a pair of platinum electrodes located at the bottom of a narrow gutter incised on the upper surface of a Perspex block. Initially, no attention was paid to where the junctions of a segment's plantar and calcaneal tributaries were located relative to the electrodes. However, when it became apparent that a segment's responses strengthened when the junctions of those major tributaries were positioned on or close to the electrodes, then the protocol was altered to take advantage of that fact. The reason the responses strengthened became clear later: positioning the junctions on the electrodes required compressing them so that they, along with the vein, fitted into the narrow gutter on the electrode block. That compression affected the cardinal valves of the tributaries and blocked the the venules carrying reflux to the microcirculation, that originated at the bases of the valves. That blockage strengthened the constrictor responses of the segment by reducing or abolishing the dilator effect NE has on the vein when it is present in the microcirculation. The fact that blocking or impeding reflux also strengthened the segment's constrictor responses to electrical stimulation was particularly significant because the concentration of NE released by electrical stimulation of the *in situ* canine saphenous vein is similar to its *in vivo* concentration [10,11] and both are comparable to the concentration of plasma NE in humans [2]. So, the evidence that impeding reflux of NE had strengthened the segment's constrictor responses supported the evidence from the bimodal response pattern (Figure 3b) that microcirculatory endogenous NE might have the venodilator potential to create varicosities in humans.

Turbulence

Turbulence amplified the volume of reflux perfusing the microcirculation of the canine lateral saphenous segment and strengthened the effect drugs present in the microcirculation had on the segment when they stimulated it through its adventitial surface. Turbulence has that amplification effect because it introduces radial components into the absolute axial velocity vector of pure laminar flow. In theory, without those components blood could not, regardless of the prevailing pressure gradient, flow from an artery into its branches or, by reflux, from a vein into its microcirculation. Turbulence is like the steering wheel in a car: without it a car, no matter how powerful, cannot change direction. Vortices and other forms of secondary flow are the physical expression of the radial components of turbulence; they act as biological mini pumps that distribute blood from an artery or a vein to their respective microcirculations. The energy for the mini pumps comes from the conversion of the shear flow or frictional energy that is released when the boundary layer of a moving blood stream weakens or loses its attachment to the endothelium at the free margins of branch points or valves, or at curves in the vascular tree, or at the downstream face of anything that roughens the endothelial surface such as plaques, tears, blood clots, endothelium denudations, etc. [12,13]. Because the level of the shear force of the blood stream on the endothelium determines the amount of energy released at the free margins and other sites, it also determines the intensity of the turbulence generated at the sites. And because the endothelium can detect the level of that shear force and correct any deviations it detects in it from the norm by releasing various endothelins, it effectively regulates and stabilizes the intensity of the turbulence that is generated at the primary branch points and that sheds distally into the roots of the first order branches of the arteries. And since the intensity of the turbulence determines the volume of blood that perfuses the microcirculation, other factors being equal, the endothelium can be said to regulate and stabilize the volume of microcirculatory flow. And because the volume of microcirculatory flow influences vascular tone through the effect of microcirculatory plasma NE, the endothelium can be said to influence vascular tone, both directly through its endothelins and indirectly through its control of the quantity of plasma NE perfusing the microcirculation.

The distributive effect of vascular turbulence is impressive. As an illustration, when monkeys were made atherosclerotic by diet, the turbulence induced by the cholesterol plaques increased flow to the microcirculation of the thoracic aortas 13-fold, from 1.3 to 17 ml/min/100gm, and 14-fold to the microcirculation of the abdominal aortas, from 2.2 to 31 ml/min/100gm. And significantly, those increases occurred without any change having taken place in the blood pressure or in the cardiac output and the flow volumes reverted to normal when a change in diet resulted in the plaques disappearing [14]. Further illustrating the distributive effect of turbulence, when flow was normal in the canine segments and their reflux channels were known to be open, the microcirculations of the segments remained visibly unstained when ink was added to the perfusate, at pressures exceeding 200mmHg. However, when turbulence was induced in the perfusate, by moving a perforated tube back and forth in the lumen of the segment, the microcirculations stained intensely at pressures of around 100 mmHg [3], and when turbulence was intensified still further by floating a length of knotted thread in the perfusate, while, at the same time, deforming the segment by gently rubbing the skin over it, not only did ink stain the microcirculation of the segment but it also stained the microcirculations of every neighboring tissue, vascular and nonvascular alike, up to about a 2cm distance from the segment [9]. Because plasma NE dilates all the pre and postcapillary vessels of the vascular and other microcirculations (see later), it was significant that skeletal muscle was one of the tissues whose vessels were stained by reflux from the vein. The significance comes from the fact it means the vascular bed of skeletal muscle is functionally part of the vascular microcirculation and consequently can be expected, pharmacologically, to dilate in response to NE. Statements to the effect that the dilatation of the skeletal muscle vascular bed by NE is exceptional is based on the mistaken belief that the bed is part of the macrocirculation.

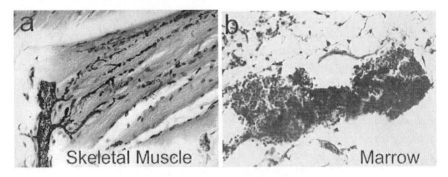

Figure 4. Photographs of (a) venules in skeletal muscle and (b) bone marrow stained with ink by reflux from a constricted canine vein segment with turbulent perfusate.

The fact that the extensive distribution of reflux just described occurred at a pressure of around 100mm Hg illustrates the fact that the Poiseuille relationship between flow and pressure does not hold when flow is turbulent.

Turbulence is a feature of the root (inlet) of all the first order branches of the conduit arteries [13]. Its effect peaks at around 2-3 times the branch diameter downstream from the branch point [15,16]. That is significant because the second order branches supplying the arterial microcirculations typically originate at about the same distance [17,18].

The first evidence I had that turbulence in the vein lumen increases reflux flow through the venous microcirculation came from experiments where *in vitro* segments occasionally developed spontaneous turbulence when they constricted in response to intralumenal NE and electrical stimulation. By increasing perfusion of the microcirculation spontaneous turbulence caused segments to dilate periodically in the course of constricting in response to bouts of random turbulence amplifying reflux perfusion of the microcirculation by NE. This mixture of constrictor followed by dilator effects caused the bimodal spike and trough pressure response patterns in Figure 3a, and, that caused segments constricting in response to electrical stimulation to dilate abruptly while they were still being stimulated (Figure 3b). Consistent with turbulence amplified reflux perfusion of the venous microcirculation being the cause of bimodal response patterns, the patterns ceased when reflux was prevented by repositioning ties on the tributaries from being distal to being proximal of the cardinal valves, in whose bases the reflux channels originated. Those latter ties will be referred to in future as close ties.

The A/V Module

The microcirculation consists of structurally isolated segments in series. Each segment services a unit called an A/V module, whose core consists of two 3-5 diameter long sections of a high pressure artery and its companion low pressure vein. The blood perfusing the arterial and venous microcirculations of an A/V module is supplied through a second order branch of the arterial section originating in the turbulent root (inlet) of the section's first order branch. The arterial and venous sections, together with their microcirculations and their adrenergic plexuses and the adrenergic plexuses of the microcirculations, form the A/V module. The entire circulation, including the heart, is composed of A/V modules, with the cardiac modules being highly modified.

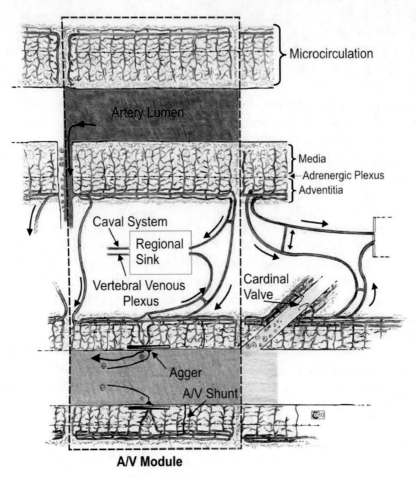

A/V Module

Figure 5. Schematic drawing illustrating a typical A/V module and the location of the cardinal valve of a tributary.

Where veins, like the canine saphenous, have no companion arteries, their microcirculations are supplied through individual unnamed small arteries, in the 150-200µ diameter range, present in the same fascial plane as the vein.

The dedicated second order blood vessels supplying the microcirculations of an A/V module originate about 2-3 primary branch diameters from the primary branch points where the dissipative effect of the physiological turbulence in the primary branches peaks and maximizes flow through the microcirculations. The second order branches divide and send third order branches to supply blood to the arterial and venous microcirculations of the A/V module. There is evidence that those third order branches further subdivide and supply possibly up to four vascular endfields in each of the twin microcirculations. The existence of those multiple endfields is believed to be the anatomical basis for the fact that pathological dilitations of the arterial and venous sections of an A/V module, viz., aneurysms and varicosities, commonly dilate asymmetrically.

Cardiac A/V Modules

The heart consists of two modified A/V modules, each containing a high pressure ventricular section and low pressure auricular section with their microcirculations and adrenergic plexuses. Like standard A/V modules, the twin microcirculations of a cardiac module are supplied by a dedicated vessel that, topologically, is a second order branch of its high pressure ventricular section. Again like the typical module, the second order branch originates in the turbulent root of the aorta, which, topologically, is a first order branch of the ventricular section. And like a typical module, the drainage of the ventricular and auricular microcirculations combine before emptying together into the lumen of the low pressure auricular section of the module. However, cardiac modules differ radically from standard modules in one critical respect. In standard modules neuronal NE and microcirculatory plasma NE act concurrently and continuously, providing their vascular sections with a stable tone, while the two NE components act successively and intermittingly in the cardiac modules, thereby causing their tone to vary continuously from very high to very low.

If, as appears, the cardiac and standard A/V modules have basically the same structure, then it is reasonable to assume that they also function in basically the same way. So, because the vascular sections of the cardiac module are highly dependent on their microcirculation to function properly, as evident from the high level of mechanical and functional crosstalk between the cardiac muscle and the cardiac microcirculation [19] and by the 100% correlation that exists between a normal heart and a normal cardiac microcirculation and a diseased microcirculation and a diseased heart, it is reasonable to assume the vascular sections of standard A/V modules have an equally high dependency on their microcirculations, not merely for nutrition but for regulatory control also.

Drainage of the A/V Module

In normal circumstances, the microcirculation of the arterial section of an A/V module drains into the postcapillary network of the microcirculation of its companion venous section. There it combines with the drainage from the microcirculation of the venous section and drains into the twin horns of a crescentic elastic structure called a valve agger (Figures 12&15). Having traversed that structure the drainage venules combine into a single 100-150μ diameter venule that drains into the base of a valve sinus of either a valve in the vein lumen or a cardinal valve in the terminal segment of a tributary. Based largely on an estimate of the number of cardinal valves versus parietal valves in the canine vein segment, up to a minimum of possibly 80% of microcirculatory drainage in a dog takes place through the cardinal valves of the tributaries. Limited observation suggests a similar proportion may apply to humans.

The A/V module changes the way it drains in two circumstances. One, when reflux is taking place and the other, when the drainage load exceeds the normal handling capacity of the drainage system. The latter may happen when arteries are atherosclerotic and, as noted, arterial microcirculatiory flow may increase 14-fold or more [14]. When the modular drainage changes it empties into a regional sink provided by the spare capacity of the postcapillary networks of every neighboring tissue between the skin and bone marrow, inclusive (Figures 4&5). From there blood drains into the caval system, preferentially, but, if that's not possible, it drains via the vertebral venous plexus and the azygos veins into the terminal segment of the vena cava [20]. Consistent with the existence of two drainage options the microcirculatory network is characterized by twin cross connected companion venules, one presumably designed to drain into the caval system and the other into the regional sink. The venules flank an artery of comparable diameter and form a triad that is iconic of the vascular [21], cardiac [19] and renal microcirculations [22], (Figure 6).

The evidence that the microcirculations of the A/V modules are interconnected through the postcapillary networks of the local vascular and non-vascular tissues means that increased levels of plasma NE in the venous microcirculation of an A/V module can, when the pressure gradients favor it, or the existence of reflux perfusion demands it, drain into the venous microcirculations of nearby A/V modules and create secondary varicosities in them (see below). Those increased plasma NE levels may, by their increased negative neurotrophic effect (see below), affect non-vascular tissues and be responsible for the structural damage sometimes exhibited by the calf muscles of patients with varicose veins [23].

A/V Shunts

The A/V module can be regarded as having a third drainage option, in the sense that it possesses A/V shunts that open when its venous microcirculation is perfused by reflux (Figures 5&21). The shunts short circuit the arterial inflow to the venous microcirculation of a module to enable the reflux responsible for opening them to be accommodated by the microcirculation. Shunts open within seconds of reflux commencing, triggered in some unknown way by the NE present in the reflux. The basis for that belief is the observation that ISO opens A/V shunts very rapidly also, but does so only when it perfuses the venous microcirculation by orthograde flow.

The Structural and Functional Independence of Modules

Figure 6 illustrates the sharp boundary and functional independence that exists between the vascular modules of the canine saphenous vein. The neighboring modules of the vein segment in Figure 6a were being perfused with a 3μM NE /ink solution and those in Figure 6b with a 50 μM ACh solution at the time of fixation. In 6a the right hand module is dilated and its microcirculation is stained by ink because its reflux channels were open when turbulence amplified the volume of reflux perfusing its microcirculation; the left hand module is constricted and its microcirculation is unstained because its reflux channels were closed off by ties, so it was stimulated only through its lumenal surface and any ink in its lumen was washed out by fixative, making the vein section appear clear. The constricted and dilated cross sections In Figure 6b were located 12mm apart at fixation in a vein segment, all of whose modules had open reflux channels. When random turbulence was induced in the segment, some modules received amplified volumes of reflux, causing thems to dilate while other modules received no amplification and they constricted in response to the relatively unopposed intralumenal effect of ACh.

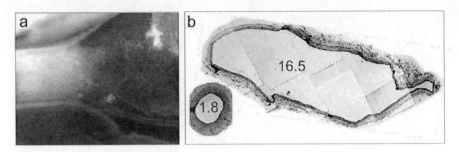

Figure 6. Figures showing (a) the sharp boundary between neighboring A/V modules and (b) two cross sections of two A/V modules, sectioned in identical planes,12mm apart in a vein perfused by ACh. The marked differences in the circumference of the two modules illustrates their potential functional independence. Figures measure the internal circumferences of the sections in arbitrary units.

The Regulatory Function of the Adrenergic Plexus and the Microcirculation

The adrenergic plexus and microcirculation of the venous section of a module are the main regulators of its tone. They stabilize the tone at a physiological level by each responding to any change in the level of activity of the other by a homeostatic change that restores any disturbed balance between the opposing effects of the two regulators.[The effect of microcirculatory plasma NE is a function of its concentration and microcirculatory flow volume, while that of neuronal NE is a function of the level of adrenergic plexus activity.] Reflecting that fact, because a varicosity is associated with an increased dilator effect of the plasma NE in the microcirculation of the affected venous module (see below),it is also associated with an increased level of activity by the adrenergic plexus of the affecterd module. The venous adrenergic plexus (VAP), like the microcirculation, is composed of functionally separate units, each regulating the tone of the venous section of a module. Bancroft may have been the first to demonstrate this functional segmentation [24]. Evidence of functional segmentation can be seen in the response of the VAP to a venous section being dilated by increased microcirculatory NE stimulation and in the physical change that occurs in the VAP of an established pathological varicosity. In the former situation, the homeostatic increase in the activity of the VAP associated with the dilated vascular section is limited to that section and does not affect the tone of the sections in the two neighboring modules, and in the latter situation, the neurones of the VAP associated with a pathological varicosity, and that segment only, becomes apoptotic.

The increased VAP activity response to increased plasma NE stimulation of a venous module mirrors what happens in the arterial side of the circulation. There the arterial adrenergic plexus (AAP) of arteriosclerotic modules displays the same type of increased segmental homeostatic response to the increased plasma NE stimulation that those modules experience (14). As a result modules of arteriosclerotic arteries display no appreciable short term dilatation in response to the increased dilator effect of microcirculatory plasma NE they experience. Evidence of homeostatic increases in adrenergic activity is also a feature of atherosclerotic cardiac disease [2,26], a condition associated with increased coronary flow and therefore with increased plasma NE stimulation of the ventricular and auricular sections of the cardiac modules [25]. Due to its clinical implications the mechanism underlying the homeostatic relationship between neuronal and plasma NE has, effectively, been investigated extensively in arteriosclerotic cardiac disease and its most important finding has been that the homeostatic increase in cardiac adrenergic activity associated with increased cardiac microcirculatory flow triggers a positive feedback loop where the increased homeostatic activity of the cardiac adrenergic plexus increases the plasma NE concentration in the coronary flow which evokes a further compensatory increase in cardiac adrenergic activity and so on. Effectively, the attempt by the cardiac adrenergic plexus to maintain the physiological balance between the opposing effects of neuronal and plasma NE generates a relentless creep in cardiac adrenergic activity that results in the concentration of cardiac plasma NE reaching toxic levels [27] that are responsible, through a negative neurotrophic effect, for lengthening the cardiomycyte sarcomeres [28], for cardiomyocyte apoptosis [29] for loss of cardiomyocyte contractility [28], and for cardiac adrenergic plexus apoptosis [30], all features that contribute to fatal dilator cardiac failure. In dealing later with the details of the pathophysiology of varicose veins the assumption will be made that the interplay between the two main regulators of venous tone also gives rise to toxic concentrations of microcirculatory plasma NE that have analogous effects on vascular smooth muscle and the venous adrenergic plexus.

The evidence that high levels of cardiac microcirculatory plasma NE are associated with structural damage highlights the fact that plasma and neuronal NE have structural as well as tonal effects on the vascular sections of the A/V modules. Neuronal NE has a positive replicative and metabolic effect that favors growth and structural integrity [31,32] while plasma NE has an opposite negative neurotrophic effect. Because increased plasma NE stimulation causes apoptosis of the adrenergic plexus [30] and because resting concentrations of plasma NE in normal subjects increases with age from 180 to250 pg/ml [33], the balance between the opposing neurotrophic effects of neuronal and plasma NE shifts, over time, in favor of plasma NE and vascular structural failure.

Evidence of the Dilator Effect of Microcirculatory NE *In Vivo*

The evidence that microcirculatory NE has a venodilator effect first emerged from experiments on the canine vein segment that showed increased reflux perfusion of the venous microcirculation by NE, caused by turbulence, dilated the segment (Figures 3&8) and blocking reflux perfusion by close ties increased the constrictor responses, to intralumenal NE and electrical stimulation, by around 50% (see below). Consistent with those findings, when pathology reduces microcirculatory flow *in vivo*, affected vessels display increased tone. A particularly striking example of that is seen in conventionally harvested venous grafts, of which almost 95% develop spasm as soon as their microcirculations are interfered with surgically, while, in contrast, grafts harvested by a new 'no-touch' technique that avoids damaging the microcirculation rarely go into spasm [4,34]. Other clinical examples of increased vascular tone being associated with interference to microcirculatory flow include Takayasu's disease and Williams Syndrome where arteries with blocked microcirculations display stenoses/coarctations [35,36] and fibrosis of the aortic microcirculation which is associated with coarctation [37]. However, the best known clinical example of increased tone being associated with blocked microcirculatory flow is the cardiospasm associated with blocked coronary microcirculatory flow.

In contrast to significant reductions in microcirculatory blood flow being associated with increased vascular tone, significant increases in microcirculatory flow caused by turbulence are associated with a loss of tone, a fact reflected clinically in arterial modules located at the site of turbulence developing aneurysms. Examples of that fact include the poststenotic dilitation (PSD) that occurs immediately downstream of a stenosis, where pathological turbulence is always a feature [38,39] and the aneurysm associated with the cervical rib syndrome where an anomalous rib deforms the lumen of the subclavian artery causing turbulence and an aneurysm downstream. However, the commonest aneurysms caused by increased microcirculatory flow, associated with pathological turbulence, are the aortic aneurysms associated with turbulence induced by cholesterol plaques.

Factors That Determine and Affect Venous Tone

Venous tone, as mentioned, is determined by the balance between the dilator effect of the plasma NE in the venous microcirculation, determined, in turn, by the level of arterial adrenergic plexus (AAP) activity, and the constrictor effect of the neuronal NE, which is determined by the level of venous adrenergic plexus (VAP) activity. Because VAP and AAP activity levels are normally independent of one another, any increase in VAP activity shifts the balance between the effects of plasma and neuronal NE on a vein in favor of neuronal NE and causes an increase in venous tone. When tone increases specific muscle bundles in the vein wall (Figures 14&15) contract and open channels originating at the bases of valves of the contracted vein to reflux. That allows venous blood, with a higher plasma NE concentration than arterial [40], perfuse the venous microcirculation by reflux and shift the balance between the two effects of neuronal and plasma NE back towards the dilator effect of plasma NE, and that, with the effect of increased plasma NE activating inhibitory presynaptic receptors of VAP activity [41], lowers the elevated venous tone to normal. As the venous tone returns to normal the specific muscle bundles responsible for opening the reflux channels relax prevent further reflux. In the canine venous segment the entire sequence of events described takes less than a minute to complete, sometimes a mere ten seconds.

When, as in varicose veins, functionally inappropriate reflux perfusion of the venous microcirculation occurs and causes a functionally inappropriate increase in the dilator effect of plasma NE then the level of VAP activity increases to counterbalance the increased dilator effect, in spite of the existence of the presynaptic inhibitory receptors that plasma NE activates when reflux is appropriate.

Because reflux perfusion of the microcirculation of a venous module is a physiological response to a rise in the module's tone, a mechanism is necessary to prevent reflux when the module's tone is normal. That mechanism is the recoil of the dense elastic fibers of the valve agger, a little known structure discussed in detail later. When for any reason, that recoil degrades, for example, due to genetic weakness of its elastic, alone or along with structural fatigue associated with prolonged standing, then episodes of inappropriate reflux occur, with each episode initiating the sequence of events just described, of which one was an increase in VAP activity that caused stretching of the elastic of the agger. That stretching helps to further degrade the recoil of the agger's already weakened elastic and, hence, facilitates an even greater increase in the volume of inappropriate reflux. In brief, functionally inappropriate reflux with its inappropriate dilator effect initiates a positive feedback loop that leads eventually to the failure of the agger and to the venous module containing the failed agger becoming varicosed. This association between a loss of elastic recoil in the vein and the development of a pathological varicosity has been recognized for some time [42,43].

For reasons that are unclear, turbulence in the vein lumen caused by such events as phlebitis, A/V fistulas, localized external pressure on the vein, etc, causes episodes of inappropriate reflux even when the recoil of the the agger experiencing the physical effect of the turbulence is normal. If the turbulence persists long enough then the episodes of reflux associated with it eventually cause the elastic of an affected agger to lose its recoil, for the reasons mentioned, and result in the venous module located at the site of the turbulence becoming pathologically varicosed. This association between turbulence and the development of pathological varicosities has also been recognized for some time [44,45].

The Role of the Vascular Microcirculation

Since its discovery in the 17th century, following Leeuwenhoek's invention of the optical microscope, the primary role of the vascular microcirculation has always been considered to be nutritional, as the original name for the network, the vasa nutritia, testifies. The more recent name for the network, the vasa vasorum, though less prescriptive, has not significantly changed the belief in the primacy of its nutritional role. However, as long ago as 1876, a German pathologist, Köester, questioned the importance of the nutritional role of the microcirculation by observing that some small venules had microcirculations considerably more dense than their apparent nutritional needs merited [46]. Then in the 1980s three morphometric studies of various arteries and veins all agreed that only a weak correlation existed between the apparent nutritional needs of the vessels and the density of their micro-circulations [47,48,49].

In view of that conclusion and the evidence of my experiments, I believe the primary role of the vascular microcirculation is, like that of the cardiac microcirculation, regulatory and based on the need for the effect of microcirculatory plasma NE to be distributed throughout the macrocirculation so it and the effect of neuronal NE can together regulate the tone of the macrocirculation and, through a joint neurotrophic effect, also regulate its structure and function. In the circumstances, the nutritional role of the microcirculation is considered to be ancillary and opportunistic, though essential.

The Renal Capsular Microcirculation

The existence of a microcirculation in the renal capsule is consistent with the primary role of the microcirculation being regulatory, in this case of the function of the kidney. The capsular microcirculation is considered to be a component of the general vascular microcirculation because it displays its the iconic vascular triad and the blood supply to its various modules originates in the physiologically turbulent inlets of first order branches of various arteries. These include the aorta, renal,renal interlobar and subdiaphragmatic [50,51].

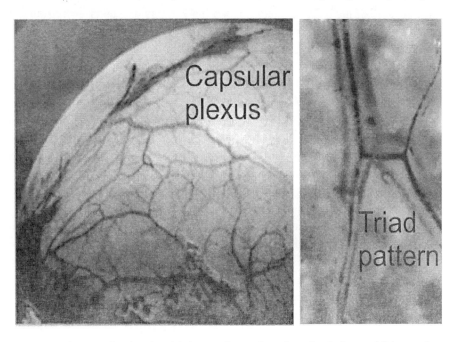

Figure 7. Photographs showing (a) the renal capsular microcirculation and (b) vascular triad.

The role of the renal capsular microcirculation (RCM) appears exceptional in being purely regulatory and lacking a significant nutritional component. That latter belief is based on the network being inappropriately located for for nutritional purposes, having a blood flow volume that appears quite insufficient to meet the apparent nutritional and metabolic needs of the renal parenchyma and the fact that the renal parenchyma has a microcirculation that appeas to be quite capable of meeting its own nutritional and metabolic needs, given each kidney receives an estimated 10% of the total cardiac output. Finally, decapsulation causes no necrotic damage to the renal structure. Evidence of the regulatory role of the RCM will be provided below.

The RCM has inflows from multiple sources presumably because it consists of modules, each originally servicing one of the embryological lobules that fuse to form the mature kidney. Fine vascular connections exist between the network and the venous vasa recta in the subcapsular plexus of the kidney [52]. The flow in those connections is minimal and what evidence there is [52] suggests it is directed centrally. By analogy with the vascular microcirculation, I suggest the fine connections are A/V shunts between the venous modules of the RCM and the renal caval drainage system. While the flow volume of the RCM is small it is not insignificant as can be seen from the fact that when a renal artery is occluded or avulsed, or a kidney is thrombosed, flow can sometimes continue in the RCM and create the tomographic cortical rim sign that clearly silhouettes the kidney [53].

The first evidence of a regulatory role by the RCM dates from the end of the 19th century when decapsulation of the kidney was introduced as an empirical, modestly successful, treatment of last resort for glomerulonephritis [54] and eclampsia [55,56]. The high morbidity and mortality of the procedure, however, led to its phasing out after only about 20 years. Today, experimental renal decapsulation confirms the regulatory role of the RCM by the fact that it is associated with changes in naturesis and diuresis [57]. (At present those changes are ascribed to alterations in the renal interstitial pressure associated with removing the capsule). Reno-vascular hypertension is believed to be one of the conditions caused by a regulatory response of the RCM. That condition is associated with turbulent flow in the aorta and/or the renal artery [58] and, therefore with pathologically increased perfusion of the RCM by plasma NE. Three features associated with renal hypertension are consistent with the condition being caused by increased microcirculatory plasma NE stimulation: one, the fact that hypertension is associated with increased renal adrenergic activity [33,59], presumably caused by a homeostatic response of the renal adrenergic network to the increased renal microcirculatory plasma NE; two, consistent with plasma NE being effectively a β_1 agonist, beta blockers are the drug of choice to treat the condition, paradoxical as that is in terms of current clinical pharmacology [60] and three, again consistent with plasma NE being an effective β_1 agonist, adrenergically mediated release of renin in the kidney is a β_1 agonist effect [61]. 'Second messenger' cAMP molecules are believed to disseminate the β_1 stimulatory effect of RCM plasma NE throughout the kidney parenchyma by way of low resistance gap junctions that are known to rapidly distribute and amplify low-level chemical signals. [62,63].

The Pharmacology of the Microcirculation

Because the macrocirculation constricts in response to intralumenal NE and dilates in response to microcirculatory NE, its different sensitivities to being stimulated by NE through the two routes cannot be compared through standard dose response curves. However, an indirect comparision of the two sensitivities suggests the macrocirculation is far more sensitive to being stimulated through its microcirculation than its lumen. The indirect comparision uses the threshold concentration at which microcirculatory ISO constricts the vein segment, which is 1ng/ml [1], as proxy for the threshold at which microcirculatory NE dilates it. On that basis the vein segment is around forty five times more sensitive to the effect of microcirculatory NE than it is to the effect of intralumenal NE. Assuming that figure is broadly correct, then because intralumenal NE vasoconstricts at 1000-1500 pg/ml, microcirculatory plasma NE with a basal concentration of around 400pg/ml [64], should be quite capable of vasodilating.

While concenirculation alone largely determines the quantitative effect a drug has when it acts intralumenally in the macrocrculatio, the effect of a drug acting via the microcirculation on the macrocirculation or bodily organs is a function of its concentration x flow x time. Consistent with that fact when turbulence was induced in a canine vein segment, perfused intralumenally with ACh, it amplified reflux flow to the microcirculations of the vein's modules, in a random manner, causing the modules' responses to differ qualitatively and quantitatively [65]. Modules whose microcirculations received little or no reflux constricted, while those whose microcirculations received significant reflux dilated in proportion to the volume of reflux they received.

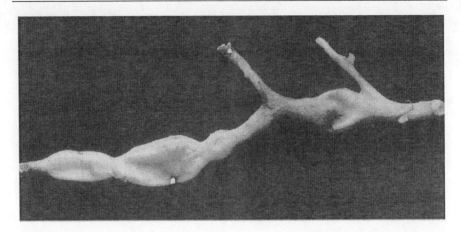

Figure 8. Photograph of a vein segment, stimulated by intralumenal ACh when its perfusate was turbulent, displaying a variety of qualitative and quatitative modular responses.

Myocardial ischemia and hyperemia illustrate how microcirculatory flow volumes alter the quantitative and qualitative effect of microcirculatory plasma NE on the cardiac modules. The ischemia is characterized by a reduction in the dilator effect of microcirculatory plasma NE, and hence by a relative increase in cardiac tone and in hypertrophy [66]. The hyperemia is characterized by an increased dilator and negative neurotrophic effect of plasma NE that is associated with cardiac dilatation, a loss of cardiac tone and and a reduction in the myocardial muscle mass.

The fact that ISO and NE have each two opposing effects on the canine segment, depending on whether they act through its microcirculation or intralumenally, provides a physical rather than a pharmacological basis for the classification of adrenergic receptors into α_1, α_2, β_1, β_2 types. The α_1/β_2 effect of NE represents its intralumenal and neuronal effects and the α_2/β_1 effect represents its microcirculatory effect. The β_1 effect of ISO corresponds to its intralumenal effect and effectively corresponds to the effect of plasma NE, the β_2 effect of ISO corresponds to the intralumenal effect NE has on the macrocirculation.This free interchangeability of effects suggests the receptors activated by NE and ISO are structurally identical. The suggestion is consistent with the theory that NE activates structurally identical receptors when generating contrasting effects during vascular smooth muscle cell contraction [67].

The experiments on the canine segment have indicated that antagonists, like agonists, change their qualitative effects depending on their route of action. So antagonists that block agonists' effects when acting by one route continue to block the different effects of the agonists when both act together by another route.However drugs that relate as agonist and antagonist when acting together by one route of stimulation do not relate when the two act by different routes [39]. The classical example of an agonist and antagonist retaining their relationship when both change their route of action and the effect of the agonist changes, is illustrated by the "paradoxical" action of beta blockers in treating angina, a constrictor event. Intralumenal beta blockers antagonize the dilator effect of intralumenal NE on epicardial coronary vessels and they continue to antagonize its effect when NE stimulates and constricts the vessels after diffusing from the pathological microcirculation those vessels develop as part of the arteriosclerotic syndrome. This "paradoxical" constrictor effect of NE on arteriosclerotic coronaries is not unique to NE: ACh [68] and serotonin [69] display this same effect. Another pharmacological concept that appears o emerge from the experiments on the canine segment is that the qualitative response of the vascular smooth muscle cell to a stimulus depends on the orientation of the major flux of the stimulus. The closer that is to the long axis of the cell the more powerful the stimulus is in contracting the cell, while the closer it is to the short axis the more powerful it is in relaxing it. By extension, a stimulus with a major flux orientated 45° to the long axis of the cell may activate the cell's receptors without eliciting any detectable response but, by altering the ratio of excitor and inhibitory receptors already activated by another stimulus may possibly alter the response to that latter stimulus [67]. That suggestion ties in with the "spare receptor" concept.

SECTION 3.

The Stenotic Constrictor Effect of Isoprenaline

Because the perfusate flow was orthograde and a competent valve prevented axial reflux at the plantar tributary junction when ISO first stenosed the canine vein segment, the search for the origin of the vessel that had transported the drug from the tributary to the site of the stenosis naturally focused on the region of the tributary junction and the nearby cardinal and ostial valves. However repeated examinations failed to detect any visible evidence of a small vessel consistently opening at any of those sites. In relation to the valves, that was not unexpected because the common belief then, as now, was that valves are cul-de-sacs. Consistent with that belief I found only one instance of a vessel opening into the sinus of a supposedly healthy valve in numerous illustrations of the structure going back to Fabricius' *De Venarum Ostiolis,* published in 1603. However, an accidental opening made into the sinus of a cardinal valve by a curved microscissors gave me the evidence I was looking for. Through the opening I saw a thin column of blood flowing, for several minutes, against gravity, from the base of the valve, across the parietal surface of the valve cusp, through the tributary junction, into the vein lumen. A subsequent SEM investigation located the opening from where the blood had issued, at the very base of the valve sinus. However, the nature of the opening varied with the tone of the vein. When it was low the opening was extremely difficult to detect (Figure 9a) because it was compressed and hidden at the bottom of surface folds thrown up by the recoil effect of the elastic of the agger, but when it was elevated, the folds were no longer there and the opening of a single venule,150-200µm wide, was clearly visible (Figure 9b).

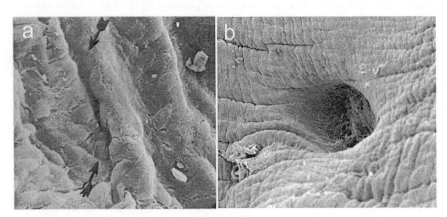

Figure 9. SEM micrographs of the bases of cardinal valves showing (a) the compressed opening of a venule, indicated by arrows, when the tone of the canine segment was normal and (b) the expanded opening of the venule when the tone was elevated.

The nature of the venular opening at the base of the valve sinus is significant in terms of function because when it is compressed it acts as a functional valve, commonly referred to as a Starling valve or resistor. Paradoxically, the compression assists the microcirculation to drain into the valve sinus while strongly resisting reflux in the opposite direction [70]. The presence of this highly effective valve is the reason, presumably, why, historically, no one could perfuse the microcirculation of a normal vein by reflux when its tone was normal or, postmortem, it was absent.

To determine if the venule seen draining into the base of the cardinal valve of the plantar tributary had been involved in the original stenotic effect of ISO, I repeatedly injected a 1ml bolus of the drug deep into the valve through a cannula (Figure 10) and, without exception, the injections stenosed the vein upstream of a competent ostial valve[39].

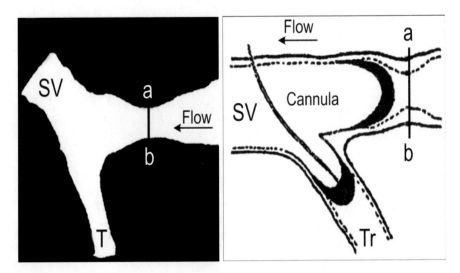

Figure 10. (a) a saphenous vein (SV) segment constricted locally, upstream of the junction of a plantar tributary (T) whose cannulated cardinal valve had been injected with ISO and (b) a diagram illustrating the injection technique and the location of the ostial valve preventing any injected drug reaching the constricted area by axial reflux from the tributary junction.

However, where the drug stenosed the segment seemed to me to be too close to the tributary junction to have been the site originally stenosed by ISO. That raises the question as to whether the ostial valve in the vein, just distal to the tributary junction, rather than the cardinal valve of the plantar tributary was involved in the original constrictor effect of ISO. That issue remains.

I have used the cannulation technique to demonstrate the effectiveness of the Starling valve mechanism in preventing reflux. I did that by injecting Methylene Blue dye into the sinus of the cardinal valve of the plantar tributary 12 times, as forcefully as possible, and recovered 92.56% (SD ±3.16) of it in the first ten ml of washout, implying the valve had prevented reflux of a minimum of around 95% of the dye injected. I performed an additional 12 injections into the distal plantar tributary itself rather than its cardinal valve, and I recovered 95.66% (SD ±3.36) of that dye [39].

THE VALVE AGGER

In veins that respond to NE stimulation, valves have two aggers; in veins that do not respond, such as some splenic veins, they have none [71]. That suggests aggers are not designed to be mere hinges connecting the valve cusps to the vein wall, as currently believed, but have some functional relationship to endogenous NE. Structurally, aggers are crescentic in form, triangular in cross section and are located along the line of attachment of the valve cusps. They are composed of dense fibro elastic..

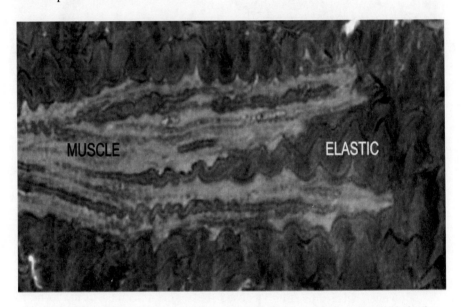

Figure 11.Micrograph showing smooth muscle inserting on the dense recoiled elastic of a valve agger.

Aggers run obliquely through the media of the vein from the adventitia to the intima at the bases of the valve sinuses. Combined drainage from the A/V modules enters the horns of the aggers before traversing them and emptying into the bases of the valve sinuses. Aggers are an essential element of the homeostatic venodilator feedback mechanism that uses reflux perfusion of the venous microcirculation with circulating plasma NE to correct elevated venous tone. Other essential elements of that mechanism are two groups of four muscles each that originate in the vein wall or the tributary wall and insert on the aggers from opposite directions so, when they contract the stretch the elastic of the aggers [65].

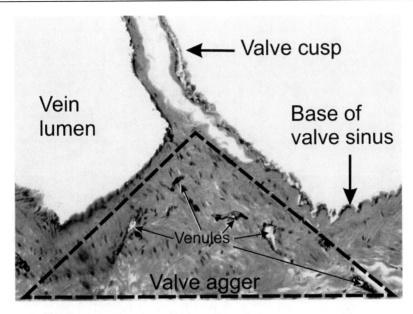

Figure 12. Micrograph of a valve agger, transversly sectioned at the base of a valve sinus and displaying sectioned drainage venules.

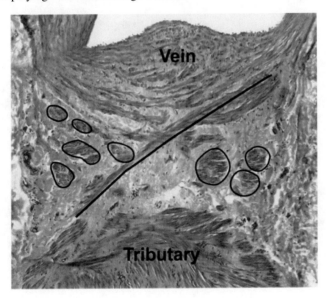

Figure 13. Micrograph showing muscle bundles projecting from a vein to the cardinal valve agger of a tributary vessel decussating in the closed angle between the vein and the tributary.

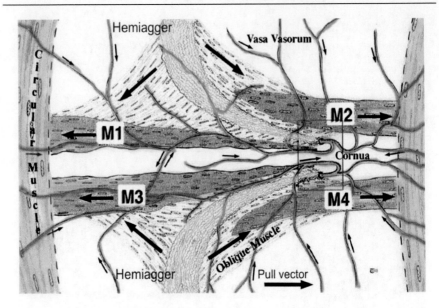

Figure 14. Schematic drawing showing four smooth muscle bundles inserting on two hemiaggers from opposing directions. Large arrows indicate the pull vector of the muscles and small arrows indicate the drainage direction of venules.

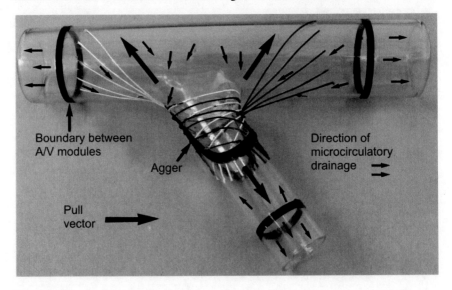

Figure 15. Photograph of a model of a cardinal valve agger showing S-formed muscle bundles, projecting on to it from a vein.

As illustrated schematically in figures 14 and 15, four muscle bundles project from the vein and/or the tributary wall and insert on the aggers of parietal and cardinal valves from opposing directions. When the venous tone is normal and the muscle bundles are relaxed, the elastic of the agger recoils and throws the base of the valve sinus into deep folds, preventing reflux, but when the venous tone rises, the muscle bundles contract and stretch the elastic of the agger thus enabling reflux to occur that lowers the venous tone and forces the drainage of an affected A/V module to be diverted into the regional sink [65]. In addition to forcing modular drainage to divert, an episode of reflux causes a number of other adjustments that   physically accommodate the volume of reflux entering the microcirculation. Two of those adjustments, the very rapid opening of A/V shunts [9] and the slower formation of intimal cushions in the arterioles of the venous microcirculation [77], greatly reduce orthograde capillary perfusion and have the potential of causing damaging hypoxia of the venous section of an affected A/V module. However because episodes of reflux normally last less than a minute, at least in the canine vein, the adjustments never cause actual hypoxic tissue damage. However, in varicose veins, when reflux is sustained, the two adjustments are directly responsible for a substantial fraction of the structural damage associated with that condition.

The Role of the Agger in Reflux

Aggers were first mentioned by French investigators in the early 19th century, who described them, among other things, as fibrous thickenings or strings at the bases of venous valves. In 1887, a German pathologist, Epstein, coined the use of the term agger, meaning a protective ridge or low wall in Latin, for what he described as a vascularised "bulge" at the base of a valve [72]. The reason he used the term, presumably, was because he was aware that Valsalva had used the same term as a metaphor for a thickening at the bases of the "great" pulmonary and aortic valves [73]. The agger has received scant attention over the years because its function has been considered to be purely passive and of little importance. That lack of attention is reflected in the absence of any reference to the structure in recent editions of Grey's Anatomy, in 11 current histology textbooks and in three popular medical dictionaries in English and several more in other languages. As far as I am aware, only three significant references have been made to the agger in recent years. One, published by a group of Bulgarian clinical anatomists [74], compared the aggers in varicose and normal veins, another was an observation by Corcos and his colleagues that aggers in varicose veins virtually disintegrate [75], and the third was a comment by Vankov, in his monograph on veins, that aggers are the most vascularised region of the vein wall [76], which is not surprising.

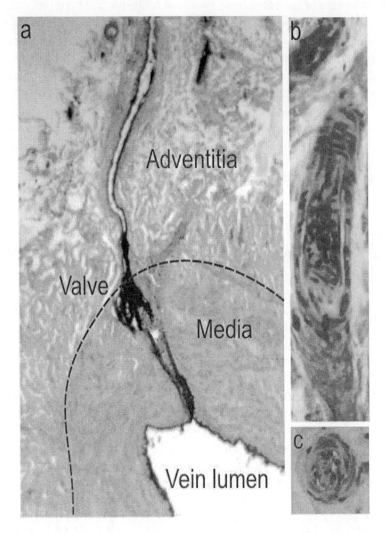

Figure 16. Micrographs showing (a) a patent A/V shunt traversing the adventitia and opening into the vein lumen. A multicusp valve, preventing reflux from the vein, is located at the medio-advential junction. (b) shows two intimal cushions in arterioles sectioned longitudinally and transversly.

The Venodilator Potency of Microcirculatory NE

The venodilator potency of microcirculatory NE in the venous segment has been estimated from the increase in strength of the segment's constrictor response to intralumenal NE and electrical stimulation following an estimated 80% reduction in reflux perfusion of the segment's microcirculation and from the increase in strength of the constrictor response to microcirculatory ISO following exhaustion of the noradrenergic stores by reserpine and guanethidine. In all situations the strength of the response increased by around 50%.

The evidence that the constrictor response to intralumenal NE and electrical stimulation increased by around 50% has come from two sources. The first is a comparision made between the responses of 57 segments with unimpeded reflux and 27 other segments with impeded reflux caused by close ties on every visible tributary of the segments regardless of size [1]. A review of the responses of the two groups showed that a range of constrictor responses that had been achieved by NE concentrations ranging between 0.1 to 0.3 µg/ml when reflux was unimpeded was achieved, when reflux was impeded, by NE concentrations ranging between 0.05 to 0.1 µg/ml. Similarly, a review of the responses of the two groups to a test electrical stimulus showed that the response made to 500 stimuli at 20Hz when reflux was unimpeded was achieved by 200-300 stimuli at the same frequency when reflux was impeded [1]. And finally, a review of all 1081 responses of the two groups to electrical stimulation found that only 13 of the 57 segments (23%) with unimpeded reflux had achieved at least one response of 80 mmHg, while 18 of the 27 segments (66%) with impeded reflux had achieved that figure.

The difference in response between segments with impeded and unimpeded reflux was unchanged when *in situ* rather than *in vitro* segments were involved [78]. That was shown by comparing the dose response curves of eleven pairs of *in situ* segments, one of each pair having unimpeded and the other impeded reflux, to 0.2, 0.6,1.5, 3.0 and 6.0 µM NE (Figure 17). The results showed that apart from the responses to 0.2 µM NE, where no significant difference was found, the responses at all other concentrations were significantly greater when reflux was impeded. In round figures, when reflux was unimpeded the responses to 0.6,1.5, 3.0 and 6.0 µM NE were, 33, 53, 87 and 126 mm Hg, respectively, but when reflux was impeded the figures rose to 49, 83, 131 and 196 mm Hg. That represents a persistent increase of around 50%.

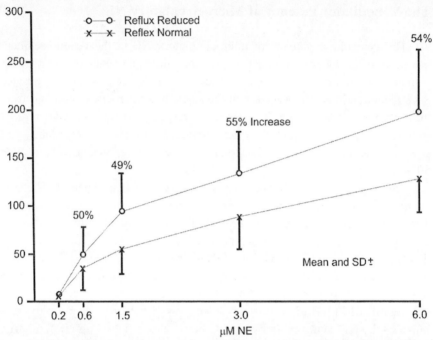

Figure 17. Dose response curves to NE when reflux was unobstructed and was reduced. It indicates that a reduction in reflux strengthened the constrictor response to NE by around 50%.

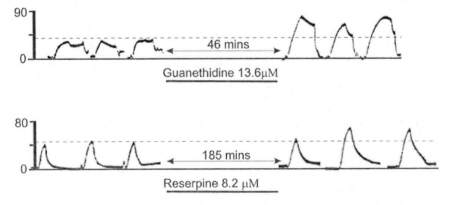

Figure 18. Records showing that exhausting the release of NE by guanethidne and reserpine increased the constrictor response of the canine vein segment to ISO by around 50% overall.

The evidence that the NE released by tonic adrenergic activity has a dilator potential comparable to that of the NE released by electrical stimulation has been provided by an experiment [39] where reserpine and guanethidine exhausted the noradrenergic stores of the canine venous segment, as evidenced by the segment ceasing to respond to electrical stimulation, and the constrictor response to micrculatory ISO increased by more than 50% sometimes (Figure 18). Apart from the fact that this experiment shows the dilator effect of NE released by tonic adrenergic activity and therefore, presumably, the dilator potential of microcirculatory NE in vivo, it eliminates the possibility that the physical effect of the close ties responsible for blocking reflux perfusion of the microcirculation in other experiments was a factor in the associated increase in the constrictor responses to NE.

In Vivo **Plasma NE Concentrations and Varicosities**

Anyone who proposes that plasma NE causes varicose veins has to explain how normal concentrations of plasma NE, at 400pg/ml, can cause any hormonal effect on a vein, given the most widely accepted view [2] that the threshold concentration for that to happen is in excess of 1000-1500 pg/ml [79], a value reached only in such restricted circumstances as extreme levels of exercise [33], or in patients suffering from myocardial infarction or pheochromocytoma. However, that threshold refers to the concentration of NE necessary for stimulating vessels of the macrocirculation intralumenally and fails to take account of the fact that veins, and presumably the vessels of the macrocirculation in general, are around 45 times more sensitive to being stimulated through their microcirculations. It also fails to take account of the fact that NE in the blood present in the lumen of the canine vein segments, about 20 minutes postmortem, has been used to create experimental varicosities (Figure 19). The concentration of that NE ranged from 590 to 1320 pg/ml, with an average of 950 pg/ml [80].

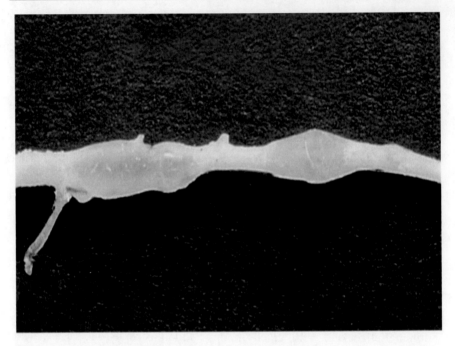

Figure 19. Photograph of varicosities on a tonically constricted canine vein segment, created by reflux of the NE present in the lumen of the segment, 20 minutes postmortem.

Varicosities Caused by Orthograde Perfusion

The only purpose of inducing turbulence when creating experimental varicosities on the canine vein was to increase the volume of reflux perfusing the microcirculations of its modules. Some may claim that a direct physical effect of turbulence on the vein wall may be responsible for varicosities, just as some claim post-stenotic dilatations (PSDs) are possibly caused by the direct physical effect of the turbulence associated with that condition [38]. However, I have created experimental varicosities, using either NE or ACh, where turbulence in the vein lumen was certainly not a factor. I achieved that result by stimulating the *in situ* cranial tibial vein via its microcirculation with either 3μM NE or 50μM Ach that had been injected forcefully, as a bolus, into the *in situ* cranial tibial artery and perfused the microcirculation of its companion vein by by orthograde flow [81].

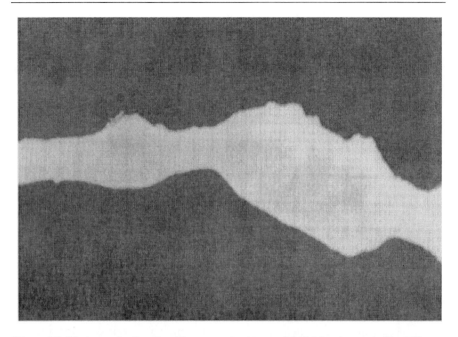

Figure 20. Photograph of varicosities on an *in situ* cranial tibial vein created by NE injected into the cranial tibial artery.

The experimental evidence that orthograde perfusion of a vein's microcirculation by NE can create varicosities on the vein may explain why patients with atherosclerosis, and, therefore, with pathological turbulence that increases perfusion of the arterial microcirculations and, presumably, of the companion venous microcirculations also, display a predisposition to varicose veins that patients with hypertension, and normal microcirculatory flow, do not [82].

The fact that ACh caused a varicosity by orthograde perfusion of a vein's microcirculation demonstrated the endothelium does not necessarily have an obligatory role in ACh relaxing smooth muscle as Furchgott and Zawadski claimed it does [83]. That claim has always been suspect because it is difficult to conceive why the endothelium would have muscarinic receptors to facilitate intralumenal ACh relaxing smooth muscle when plasma and red blood cells contain a range of specific and non specific esterases to seemingly ensure it does not do so, and when, in addition vascular beds in general lack cholinergic innervation [84]. When reviewed in the light of the information now available on the microcirculation, the most striking feature of Furchgott and Zawadski's experiment, famous for leading to the discovery of nitric oxide, was that ACh only relaxed the smooth muscle of an aortic strip when its concentration was very low. Given the exceptionally high sensitivity of vascular smooth muscle to drugs stimulating it through diffusion from a microcirculation, that fact immediately suggests ACh may have relaxed the aortic smooth muscle by stimulating it through its microcirculation. The fact that ACh failed to relax the muscle when the endothelium of the aortic strip had been abraded could be explained by the fact that when the abraded endothelium had plugged the primary branches of the strip and prevented ACh reaching the microcirculation. That possibility is given credence by the fact that photographs display patent primary branch openings in the aortic strip before the endothelium was abraded but none afterwards.

Arterial Dilitation Caused by Microcirculatory NE

When a bolus of NE was injected rapidly into *in situ* cranial tibial arteries it caused a mixture of berry aneurysms, segmental dilatations and coarctations [81]. The belief is that this was due to the rapid injections having induced randomly located turbulence that caused variable amplification of orthograde perfusion of randomly located microcirculations of the arteries, which resulted in random variable responses to NE by the modules of the arteries.

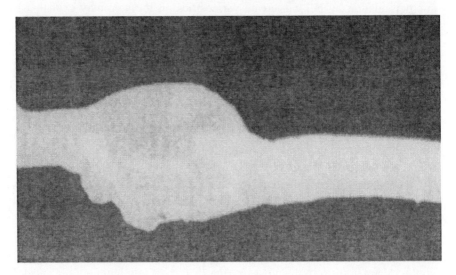

Figure 21. Photograph of a berry aneurysm on an *in situ* cranial tibial artery created by NE.

SECTION 4.

Validation

This section aims to validate the hypothesis that varicose veins result from segmental vasoregulatory failures of the venous microcirculation. It does it in two ways, by describing how the segmental failures cause varicosities, and by demonstrating that the findings associated with experimental varicosities match those found in pathological varicosities in detail or provide a credible explanation of how they probably develop.

Reflux perfusion of the venous microcirculation of an A/V module is appropriate only when the venous tone is elevated. A vein prevents it happening when the tone is normal by the Starling valve mechanism, which depends for its effectiveness on the recoil of the dense elastic of the valve agger. The failure of the agger's recoil allows inappropriate reflux occur even when the venous tone is normal and is believed to be the index event that triggers the development of a varicosity in the module associated with the failed agger. In primary varicose veins the agger's failure is believed to be structural, while in the case of secondary varicose veins it is believed to be functional and due, for some unknown reason, to turbulence induced by, e.g., A/V fistulas, phlebitis, vein deformation, etc. The failure of an agger in primary varicose veins is believed to be due to factors like structural fatigue caused by prolonged standing, genetically weak elastic, high relaxin levels in pregnancy, gender and racial factors, etc. At first the degree of failure of an agger and the volume of the associated inappropriate reflux are minimal and the situation is reversible. However if the factor responsible for causing the agger failure persists then episodes of inappropriate reflux keep on recurring, each one triggering the homeostatic response sequence described earlier, which in the dog lasts less than a minute, and involves the venous adrenergic plexus (VAP) causing a compensatory smooth muscle contraction that has the collateral effect of stretching the elastic of the failing agger. The predictable effects of this are an increasing loss of elastic recoil of the failing agger and hypertrophy of the smooth muscle that makes a varicosity radix palpable before it becomes visible [85].

The increase in size displayed by the varicosity radix is not simply due to a failure of its muscle which, as noted, hypertrophies initially, but is caused by the increased plasma NE dilator effect caused by the spiral in the volume of inappropriate reflux with its increasing concentrations of plasma NE, caused by the positive feedback loop triggered by increased VAP activity. In addition to the malign effect of that spiral, the increasing curvature of the developing varicosity radix increases local turbulence that adds further to the volume of inappropriate reflux perfusing the microcirculation of the varicosity, and further increasing the dilator effect of the microcirculatory NE on the varicosity. The evidence of this gradual increase in the volume of inappropriate reflux associated with a developing varicosity radix is well established [86].

In terms of their potential to cause damage, the most significant adjustments associated with developing pathological human varicosities are the opening of A/V shunts [87] and the formation of arteriolar intimal cushions [88]. The experimental varicosities showed those same adjustments occurring in response to reflux perfusion of the venous microcirculation by NE. There the shunts opened within seconds of a single bout of reflux occurring [9], while the intimal cushions formed within a maximum of 6 hours following several bouts of reflux {89] (Figure 16). The predictable consequence of those two changes is a significant reduction in orthograde capillary perfusion of the venous microcirculation. While that would be of little consequence when an episode of reflux is shortlived, when bouts of reflux occur repeatedly or are persistent the consequences are serious, because they cause hypoxic damage of the varicosed venous section of the affected A/V module, and its associated tissues such as the fascial coats of the section that normally limit its dilatation. Needle probes [90] and positron emission tomography [91] have provided direct evidence of the chronic hypoxia, while changes in the enzyme profile in varicose veins from aerobic towards anerobic [92,93], and an early loss of oxidative enzymes by the cristae of the mitochondria of smooth muscle in the varicosity wall [94] have provided indirect evidence of its existence. Other predictable consequences of chronic tissue hypoxia that are evident in pathological varicosities [91,95,96] include degeneration of the collagen, elastic and smooth muscle components of the vein wall.

If developing pathological varicosities are associated with increasing volumes of inappropriate reflux and a relentless spiral in the concentration of the plasma NE present in the reflux then a point eventually arrives where the effect of plasma NE becomes demonstrably toxic. Based on what occurs in a failing heart when plasma NE levels become toxic [29] one of the expected consequences of a toxic plasma concentration in a vein would be apoptosis of its adrenergic plexus. And that in fact is a recognized feature of pathological varicosities [97]. That apoptosis has serious consequences because it leads to the lessening of the positive neurotrophic, replicative and metabolic influence of neuronal NE on the varicosity wall [31,32]. And again based on what is found in the pathological heart [27,28], other likely consequences of toxic levels of plasma NE stimulation that are known to occur in pathological varcosities, include apoptosis of the venous smooth muscle with fibrous replacement. Degeneration of the valve agger [75] and the loss of valve competency would be further expected consequences of the effects of an increased negative neurotrophic NE influence and chronic hypoxia on the collagen in a varicosity.

Hemosiderotic staining of the skin in the gaiter region is a recognized feature of chronic varicose veins. The phenomenon is usually explained as being caused by the seepage of red blood cells through damaged postcapillaries and their subsequent breakdown in the surrounding tissues. However it is possible the cells may have extravasated through a structurally sound postcapillary venule given the evidence of a large fenestration, nearly 12μm across in its main axis, being found in an adventitial venule, that had experienced several bouts of experimental reflux perfusion [77].

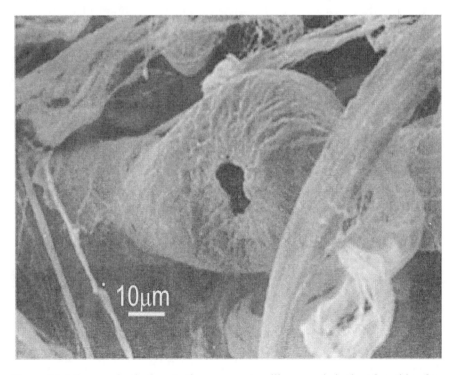

Figure 22. Micrograph of a fenestration on a postcapillary venule in the adventitia of a vein segment.

The Multiplication of Varicosities

One of the more distressing features of varicose veins is their unfailing tendency to multiply. I believe that multiplication effect is caused by a collateral effect of the reflux associated with the formation of a varicosity. That reflux necessarily drains into the regional sink from the varicosed module. From that sink it is structurally possible, if the pressure gradients favor it, for the reflux to perfuse the postcapillary networks of neighboring venous modules. Assuming that it does so, then the reflux acts as secondary reflux in the recipient module and triggers the same sequence of changes as it has triggered in the donor venous module. That means it triggers the opening of A/V shunts and the formation of intimal cushions in the microcirculation of the recipient module, with all the pathological consequences that has.

Consistent with that analysis, and keeping in mind that most primary reflux occurs through the cardinal valves of tributaries, it is significant that when, empirically, close ties were placed on the tributaries of pathological varicosities, close to their junctions, and therefore blocking further reflux to the varicosities, the tendency for secondary varicosities to occur decreased [98], presumably because secondary reflux perfusion of neighboring venous modules via the regional sink ceased.

Therapeutic Options

Ideally the time to treat varicosities is when they are at the radicular stage and their smooth muscle is hypertrophied, making them palpable as firm berry–like structures [85]. Given the therapeutic effectiveness of adrenergic blockade in many conditions believed to be caused by increased microcirculatory plasma NE stimulation [58], it is possible that a local application of some form of adrenergic blocker cream or ointment to the skin over the varicosity radix might reverse or, at least, stabilize it. In addition if the index event of varicose veins is a loss of elastic recoil in the agger then the use of elastic support wear at the first indication of a varicosity would appear to be very desirable.

However, on the basis of the available information, when a varicosity is firmly established, a rational surgical alternative treatment could be the placing of a close surgical tie on the nearest tributary to the varicosity, given that the most likely origin of the venule trnaporting the reflux responsible for the varicosity is at the base of the cardinal valve of that tributary. Should those ties be successful in blocking the reflux responsible for the varicosity then then not only would that reduce the formation of secondary varicosities [98] but it would also abolish the effect reflux NE has of opening A/V shunts and causing the formation of arteriolar intimal cushions in the primary varicosity. That, in theory, should help to reoxgenate the hypoxic issues of the varicosity and deliver other possible benign consequences that can only be speculated on. In reference to the present preference for schlerotherapy it is possible that combining that form of treatment with close tributary ties might have a therapeutic benefit greater than would be anticipated of a simple additive effect.

SECTION 5.

The Bipolar Nature of the NE Stimulus

At first glance, it seems to make little sense, in terms of efficiency and economy, for NE to have two potent cross inhibitory effects on vascular smooth muscle and other tissues. However, there are a number of reasons why this conflict exists. The first is that neuronal NE and plasma NE cause their effects by diffusing from different sources in the cardiovascular and other systems, viz., the adrenergic plexuses and the microcirculations, and, consequently, they generate different 4D-diffusion patterns [99,100] that necessarily have different effects on their target tissues, whose responses reflect the precise nature of the patterns [65]. The second is that all tissues are biological chemosensors, and consequently, their primary stimulus, NE or ACh, like all primary stimuli investigated to date, possesses two components that display cross inhibitory effects [101,102]. The two components are commonly referred to as excitor and lateral inhibitory, with the latter being the most potent physiological modulator of the former [103].

The third reason the NE stimulus has two contrasting effects is because it is a biological signal and all signals deliver information in the form of 4-D patterns that need contrast for the information they carry to be detected and retrieved. That universal principle is illustrated by the familiar barcode signal that delivers information in the form of a pattern of lines of varying thickness and spacing. However for that information to be detected and retrieved the lines need to be printed on a background of a different color to themselves. Lines printed on a background of similar color still contain information but it cannot be retrieved. Photographers are particularly aware of this need for contrast, but are also aware that the level or balance of contrast is as important as its existence: too much can be as bad as too little in the making of a good photograph. In that context, the homeostatic increase in the levels of adrenergic plexus activity evoked by increased effects of microcirculatory plasma NE can be viewed as being an attempt by the body to maintain the optimum contrast or balance possible between the excitor and inhibitory effects of the NE stimulus under changing circumstances.

The Roles of Neuronal and Plasma NE in Smooith Muscle Contraction

The specific reason the NE stimulus needs or has two components in the case of smooth muscle cell (SMC) stimulation is the cell needs the two different components to be able to relax as well as contract. Basically, without plasma NE the cell cannot relax and without neuronal NE it cannot contract. To understand how these two roles of NE interact during smooth muscle contraction requires some understanding of the structure of the SMC and its contraction mechanism. There is no consensus on either of these at present but I believe a plausible and internally coherent explanation of them is possible [58,67], that is based on the extensive information now available on the structure of the cell [104,105] and on extrapolation from the way skeletal muscle and mobile non-muscle cells, like leucocytes, contract.

The Roles of NE in Smooth Muscle Contraction

The unit of contraction of the spindle shaped SMC is the myofibril, a hollow conical structure, filled with contractile inclusions and measuring a half cell in length. The cell contains two interdigitated stacks of t myofibrils, each one occupying an estimated 70-80% of the length of the cell. All the myofibrils are crosslinked through cytoplamic dense bodies (CDBs), the functional equivalents of Z-discs in skeletal muscle [106] that subdivide the myofilaments of the myofibril into 2μm long sarcomeres [107]. The apical ends of the myofibrils are attached to the cell membrane of the narrow polar ends of the SMC and their expanded bases are attached to the membrane of the wide midsection of the cell. In a cell with a long /short axis ratio of 50%, the estimated apical angle of the myofibril is less than 2°. Relative to the long axis of the cell, the apex and base of a myofibril are displaced 180° radially, which means myofibrils generate torque and become coiled as they contract. That is a critical feature because it means the cell rotates as it shortens. That rotation is responsible for continuously changing the cohorts of the cell's receptors being exposed to the polarized fluxes of the diffusion patterns of neuronal and plasma NE, that are believed to be orientated in circular vascular smooth muscle with the long and short axes of the SMC respectively.

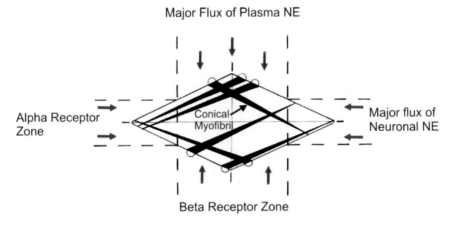

Figure 23. Diagram of a smooth muscle cell visualizing some of the concepts mentioned in the text.

Based on some assumptions and taking into account how membrane receptors are distributed on sensors like the retina and the tympanic membrane, and on unicellular organisms, [108,109], the depolarizing α_1 (β_2) and polarizing β_1 (α_2) adrenoreceptors of the SMC are believed to be segregated into four domains on the cell membrane, with two α_1 (β_2) domains occupying and being centered on the polar ends of the cell and two β_1 (α_2) domains, occupying the middle of the cell and meeting along the equator. Again, extrapolating from various sensory systems, the membrane receptors are believed to form a continuum, with the most powerful depolarizing receptors being located at the two apices of the SMC and the most powerful polarizing ones being located along the equator. When viewed *en face* along the long axis of the cell that distribution displays the 'ON'-center, 'OFF'-inhibitory surround pattern that characterizes so many sensory systems, including, in particular, the retina [110,111]. Based on the manner leucocytes and other mobile non-muscle cells decorate the myofilaments of their conical myofibrils with receptors [67] each myofilament of a SMC myofibril is believed to be decorated with two structurally identical adrenoreceptors, one at either end. It is speculated that a myofilament receives a signal to shorten when the α_1 (β_2) receptor at its apical end is activated by neuronal NE, and a signal to lengthen when the β_1,(α_2) receptor at its base is activated by plasma NE. The balance of effect between the responses to the two signals determines the length of the myofilament, and scaling up, determines the response of the SMC and blood vessels to the total NE stimulus.

Besides being responsible for activating continually changing cohorts of membrane adrenoreceptors, the two components of the NE stimulus play a second distinctive role in the smooth muscle contraction process. The need for them to play that role arises from the nature of the contraction process which involves recruiting, contracting and then removing activation from continuously changing cohorts of myofibrils during the contraction process. The cohorts are continuously introduced to the contraction process by the rotation of the SMC exposing continually changing populations of orthogonally projecting membrane receptors [112] to the two polarized NE stimuli. That arrangement implies the activated receptors of contracted myofibrils cease being activated as the cell rotates and unactivated receptors of other myofibrils become activated. Based on what appears to happen in skeletal muscle contraction, one might expect that the contracted myofibrils of the SMC would relax once their receptors are no longer activated, but that doesn't happen because of a mechanism termed "latch" which prevents it and, preserves the tension generated by the contracted myofibrils when their receptors cease being activated. Effectively, the latch mechanism freezes the actin overlap when, as happens in SMC contraction, the myosin responsible for creating the overlap is translocated along with mitochondria, SER and other contractile components from a contracted myofibril to another myofirbril due to contract shortly [113]. The latch mechanism involves the two components of the NE stimulus in phosphorylating and dephosphorylating a small regulatory chain attached to the soluble, mobile myosin of the SMC [114,115]. Neuronal NE dephosphorylates the chain and creates latchbridges (crossbridges) that maintain the actin overlap while plasma NE phosphorylates the chain and releases latchbridges and decreases the actin overlap. The balance between the two effects determines the length of a myofibril, and, scaling up, vascular tone. The balance continually adjusts to changes in the strength of the two components of the NE stimulus but normally the balance favors neuronal NE and contraction. Anything that reduces the amount of plasma NE perfusing the microcirculation of a vascular module shifts the balance in favor of contraction and anything that increases it shifts the balance in favor of relaxation. Latchbridges are virtually permanent structures that can only be released by plasma NE stimulation. Mere withdrawal of the neuronal

NE stimulus is not sufficient to release latchbridges, hence the reason stenoses are permanent features once they occur on loss of plasma NE stimulation. Based on the intrlumenal pressure vascular surgeons need to use to overcome the venospasm of coronary bypass grafts harvested in the traditional manner, it can require an intralumenal pressure of up to 300 mmHg to physically overcome the effect of latchbridges and dilate a spastic vessel. Under-standably, standard systolic pressures are never strong enough to do that, so arterial stenoses and coarctations are permanent once formed.

Cardiac contraction is believed to involve a modified latch mechanism where the two components of the NE stimulus act separately and successively. By doing so each component in turn is free to display its full potential to increase and decrease the tone of the cardiac modules. Systole displays the the full potential of neuronal NE and diastole the full potential of plasma NE..

Contraction in the Microcirculation

Contraction by the SMCs of the microcirculation involves the same mechanism as the SMCs in the macrocirculation. However while the neuronal NE component is provided by the the adrenergic plexus of the micro-circulation, as it is in the macrocirculation, the relaxing plasma NE component, unlike the macrocirculation, is provided by the intralumenal effect of the NE in the microcirculation. That latter fact is reflected in the fact that exogenous NE has a dilator effect on the microcirculation, as the porcine microcirculation,[116], the coronary microcirculation [67,117,] and the venules of the perfused canine segment all testify [9]. The reason NE dilates the vascular bed of skeletal muscle [2] is because it is part of the general microcirculatory network, as shown by the fact that it is part of the regional sink that drains the A/V modules when reflux occurs (Figure 4).

Despite their large size, the epicardial coronary vessels form part of the vascular microcirculation and, because of that they have no microcirculation when they are healthy and dilate in response to intralumenal NE [117]. However when they become atherosclerotic the epicardials develop a pathological microcirculation and then they respond to stimulation as if they are part of the macrocirculation. So, just as pathological turbulence in the macrocirculation proper increases flow to its microcirculation, pathological turbulence induced by cholesterol plaques in the coronary vessels increases perfusion of their pathological microcirculation [25, 118]. And in the same way as the intralumenal effect of NE on the macrocirculation changes qualitatively from constrictor to dilator when it stimulates the macrocirculation through release from its microcirculation, so the dilator effect of NE on the coronary vessels changes into constrictor when the drug stimulates the vessels through diffusion from their pathological microcirculation. In so far as NE does that it copies the effects of Ach [68] and serotonin [69] both of which have been shown to dilate healthy coronaries but constrict atherosclerotic ones.

The Role of the General Microcirculation

It is is assumed that the concept of the two component nature of the NE stimulus is a valid one, then any cell, or tissue or organ innervated by the sympathetic system depends on simultaneous stimulation by plasma NEand neuronal NE to function roperly. That, in effect, means plasma NE has a functional importance that is not recognized at present and it provides a rationale for the otherwise difficult to explain fact that large highly vascularised organs like the kidney and the liver have capsular microcirculations that appear inadequate and unnecessary to service their needs for oxygenated blood and nutrition. Interestingly, both the liver, in the case of cirrhosis, [119] and the kidney, in the case of hypertension [59], display evidence of increased adrenergic activity, a fact that is consistent with both conditions being associated with and, as has been proposed [58], caused by, increased microcirculatory plasma NE stimulation.

CONCLUSION

This chapter has offered a novel perspective on the etiology of varicose veins, claiming the condition is caused by structurally normal veins responding actively and appropriately to pathological levels of dilator feedback stimulation caused by plasma NE diffusing from isolated segments of the venous microcirculation. Assuming that is a orrect interpretation of the experimental and clinical data then a non-surgical therapeutic approach to the treatment of varicose veins may be possible. Given the skin has direct, unvalved vascular connections with the venous microcirculation, one possible avenue of treatment that might be is the use of catecholamine blocking agents applied in the form of a cream or ointment to the skin over the varicosity. Another therapeutic approach suggested by the findings of this chapter is the use of close surgical ties to reduce the tendency of varicosities to multiply. The procedure should, in theory, have the effect of closing down the open A/V shunts in varicosities and of resolving the arteriolar intimal cushions responsible for the low tissue pO2 associated with varicosities. Should they have that effect then the resulting restoration of a normal tissue pO2 would surely prevent the formation of the skin ulcers associated with chronic varicosities.

Another apparent finding of this chapter is that a varicosity is well established and irreversible when it is visibly, as distinct from palpably, detectable. In the circumstances patients have a reason to be encouraged to use elastic supports or avail of some pharmacological or surgical remedy at an earlier stage than is currently the norm.

In addition to its primary findings the chapter has offered a new paradigm of the vascular circulation that may help to elucidate the etiology and improve the treatment of a variety of common cardiovascular conditions. It has also introduced the concept of the primary role of the microcirculation being regulatory rather than nutritional or metabolic, thus enhancing its importance. The chapter has offered a possible physical basis for the pharmacological classification of receptors and drugs into their various alpha and beta types, a fact that may help to explain and remove a number of current pharmacological paradoxes. Finally the chapter has called circulating plasma NE in from the cold.

REFERENCES

[1]   Crotty TP. Fluidic blood vessel control – a new concept. *Ir J Med Sci*, 1969; Series VII(2): 311-315.

[2]   Esler M, Jennings G, Lambert G, Meredith I, Horne M, Eisenhoffer G. Overflow of catecholamine neurotransmitter to the circulation: source, fate and functions. *Physiological Rev*, 1990; 70:963-984.

[3]   Crotty TP. The path of retrograde flow from the lumen of the lateral saphenous vein of the dog to its vasa vasorum. *Microvascular Res,* 1989; 37: 119-122.

[4]   Driefaldt M, Souza DS, Loesch A, Muddle JR, Karlsson MG, Filbey D, Bodin L, Norgren L, Dashwood MR. The no-touch harvesting technique for vein grafts in coronary artery bypass surgery preserves an intact vasa vasorum. *J Thor Cardiovasc Surg*. DOI: 10 1016/j.jtcvs. 2010.02.005l.

[5] Bergan JJ, Pascarella L, Schmis-Schönbein GW. Pathogenesis of primary chronic venous disease: insights from animal models of venous hypertension. *J Vasc Surg,* 2008; 47(1):183-192.

[6] Burnand KG, Clementson G, Whimster I, Gaunt G, Browse NL. The effect of sustained venous hypertension on the skin capillaries of the canine hindlimb. *Br J Surg,* 1982; 69:41-44.

[7] Bradshaw W. Fluidics. *LIFE* (Atlantic Ed) 1967; 10:54-57.

[8] Crotty TP, Hall WJ, Sheehan JD. A study of perfused isolated dog saphenous vein. *Ir J Med Sci.* 1971; 140(7):05-315.

[9] Crotty TP. An investigation of the vasa venarum in a canine vein using radial reflux perfusion. *Phlebology* 1995; 10:12-18.

[10] Muldoon SM, Tyce GM, Moyer TP, Rorie DK. Measurement of endogenous norepinephrine overflow from canine saphenous vein. *Am J Physiol* 1979; 236:H263-267.

[11] Vanhoutte PM, Coen EP, De Ridder WJ, Vanbeuren TJ. Evoked release of endogenous norepinephrine in the canine saphenous vein. *Circ Res* 1979; 45:608-614.

[12] Grass AJ, Stuart AJ, Mansour-Tehrani M. Vortical structures and coherent motion in turbulent flow over smooth and rough boundaries. *Phil Trans R Soc Lond* (A). 1991; 336:36-65.

[13] Krovetz LJ. The effect of vessel branching on haemodynamic stability. *Phys Med Biol* 1965; 10:417-427.

[14] Heistad DD, Armstrong, Ml, Marcus ML. Hyperemia of the aortic wall in atherosclerotic monkeys. *Circ Res* 1981; 48(5):669-675.

[15] Palmer AA. Hemodynamics of the Microcirculation. In: *Stehbens WE. Haemodynamics and the Blood Vessel Wall.* Springfield, Ill: Charles C Thomas; 1979. p157-178.

[16] Anderson ABC. Metastable jet-tone states of jets from sharp-edged, circular, pipe-like orifices. *J Acoustical Soc Am* 1955; 27:13-21.

[17] Baker SGE, Martin JF. Role of the adventitia in atherogenesis: arterial wall vasa vasorum. In: Woodford FP, Davignon J, Sniderman A, eds. Atherosclerosis X. *Proceedings of the 10th International Symposium on Atherosclerosis.* Amsterdam: Elsevier BV; 1995. p926-931.

[18] Schönenberger F, Müller A. Über die Vaskularisation der Rinderaortenwand. *Helvet Physiol et Pharmacol Acta,* 1960; 18:136.

[19] Westerhof N, Boer C, Lamberts RR, Sipkema P. Cross-talk between cardiac muscle and coronary musculature. *Physiol Rev,* 2006; 86:1263-1308.

[20] Batson OV. The function of the vertebral veins and their role in the spread of metastases. *Ann Surg*, 1940; 112:138-149.

[21] Vio A, Gozzetti G, Reggiani G, Platania A. On the distribution of vasa vasorum in the main arteries and veins. *Angiologica*, 1964; 1:357-382.

[22] Crotty TP. Homœopathy and homeostasis in the vascular system. Part 2. *Homœopathic J*, 1989; 78:127-148.

[23] Makitie J. Muscle changes in patients with varicose veins. *Acta Pathol Microbiol Scand (A)*. 1977; 85:864-68.

[24] Bancroft FW. The venomotor nerves of the hindlimb. *Am J Physiol*, 1898; 1:477-485.

[25] Heistad DD, Armstrong ML. Blood flow through vasa vasorum of coronary arteries in atherosclerotic monkeys. *Arteriosclerosis* 1986; 6:326-31.

[26] Bristow MR. Beta-adrenergic receptor blockade in chronic heart failure. *Circ*, 2000;101:558-569.

[27] Mann DL, Bristow MR. Mechanisms and models in heart failure. The biomechanical model and beyond. *Circulation*, 2005; 111:2837-2849.

[28] Sonnenblick EH. Myocardial ultrastructure in the normal and failing heart. In: Braunwald E, editor. *The Myocardium: failure and infarction*. NY: HP publishing Co., Inc, 1974 p3-13.

[29] Communal C, Singh K, Pimental DR, Colucci WS. Norepinephrine stimulates apoptosis in adult rat ventricular myocytes by activation of β-adrenergic pathway. *Circulation*, 1998; 98:1329-1334.

[30] Braunwald E. The autonomic nervous system in heart failure. In: Braunwald E. editor *The Myocardium: failure and infarction*. NY: HP Publishing Co., Inc; 1974; 59-69.

[31] Todd ME. Trophic interactions between rat nerves and blood vessels in denervated peripheral arteries in anterior eye chamber transplants. *Circ Res*, 1986;58: 641-652.

[32] Bevan RD. Trophic effects of peripheral adrenergic nerves on vascular structure. In: Folkow B, Norlander M, Strauer B-E, Wikstrand J, eds. *Hypertension – pathophysiology and clinical implications of early structural changes*. Mölndal, Sweden; AB Hässl, 1985, p.44-58.

[33] Goldstein DS. Plasma catecholamines and essential hypertension: an analytical review. *Hypertension*, 1983;5: 86-99.

[34] Souza DSR, Bomfin V, Skoglund H, Dashwood ML, Borowiec JW, Bodin L et al. Early high patency of saphenous vein graft for coronary artery bypass harvested with surrounding tissue. *Ann Thoracic Surg*, 2001; 71: 797-800.

[35] Hall S, Barr W, Lie JT, Stanson AW, Kazmier, Hunder GG. Takayasu arteritis. A study of 32 North Americans. *Medicine* (Baltimore) 1985; 64:89-99.

[36] Arrington C, Tristani-Firouzi M, Puchalski M. Rapid progression of long-segment coarctation in a patient with William's syndrome. *Cardiol Young*, 2005; 15: 312-314.

[37] Funata N, Tanaka M, Hirokawa K. Coarctation of the abdominal aorta - case report with autopsy. *Acta Pathol Jpn*, 1981; 31:117-127.

[38] Roach MR. Hemodynamic factors in arterial stenosis and postenotic dilatation. In: Stebhens WE editor. *Hemodynamics and the Blood Vessel Wall*. Springfield, Ill; Charles C Thomas, 1979; 439-464.

[39] Crotty TP. The vasa vasorum and the paradox of beta-blocker therapy. *Medical Hypotheses*, 1992;37:191-197.

[40] Altman Pl, Dittmer DS editors. *Blood and Other Body Fluids*. Washington DC: Federation of American Societies for Experimental Biology;1961.

[41] Dixon WR, Mosimann WF, Weiner N. The role of presynaptic feedback mechanisms in regulation of norepinephrine release by nerve stimulation, *J Pharm Exp Ther*, 1978;209:196-204.

[42] Clarke H, Smith SRG, Vasdekis SN, Hobbs JT, Nicolaides AN. Role of venous elasticity in the development of varicose veins. *Br J Surg*, 1989; 76: 577-580.

[43] Shields DA, Andaz SK, Sarin S, Scurr JH, Coleridge Smith PD. Plasma elastase in venous disease. *Br J Surg*, 1994; 81: 1496-1499.

[44] Kline AL, Byrne P. Turbulence as a factor in the aetiology of varicose veins. *Br J Surg*, 1972; 59:915.

[45] Fegan WG. Varicose veins: the 'bob-sleigh' theory. *Phlebology*, 1993; 8:142-144.

[46] Köester W. Endarteritis u. arteritis. *Berl Klin Wochenschr*, 1876; 13:454.

[47] McGeachie J, Campbell P, Simpson S, Prendergast F. Arterial vasa vasorum: a quantitative study in the rat. *J Anat*, 1982; 134:193-197.

[48] Liszczak TM, Black P McL, Varsos VG, Zervas NT. The microcirculations of cerebral arteries. A morphologic and morphometric examination of the major canine cerebral arteries. *Am J Anat*, 1984; 170:223-232.

[49] Heistad DD, Armstrong ML, Amundsen S. Blood flow through vasa vasorum in arteries and veins: effects of luminal PO_2 . *Am J Physiol*, 1986; 250:H434-442.

[50] Anson BJ, McVay C., eds. *Surgical Anatomy*. 6th ed. Philadelphia, Pa: WB Saunders; 1984.

[51] Kurzidim,MH, Oeschger DM, Sasse D. Studies on the vasa vasorum of the human renal artery. *Ann Anat*, 1999;181: 223-227.

[52] Barger AC, Herd JA. The renal circulation. *NEJM*, 1971;284(9):482-489.

[53] Hann L, Pfister RC. Renal subcapsular rim sign: new etiologies and pathogenesis. *AJR*, 1982;138: 51-54.

[54] Edebohls GM. Renal decapsulation for chronic Bright's disease. *Medical Record* (NY),1903;63:481-491.

[55] Galabin A, Blacker G. The Practice of Midwifery. London: J&A Churchill; 1910.

[56] Kehrer E. Die nierendekapsulation bei eclampsie. *Z Gyn Urol* 1909;11:111-25.

[57] Khraibi AA, Knox FG. Effects of acute renal decapsulation on pressure naturesis in SHR and WKY rats. *Am J Physiol*, 1989;257:785-789.

[58] Crotty TP. The role of plasma noradrenaline in health and disease. *Bioscience Hypotheses,* 2008;1:235-242.

[59] Mancia G, Seravalle G, Grassi G. Sympathetic neural mechanisms in the pathogenesis of human hypertension. First Virtual Congress of Cardiology. *htpp://www.fac.org.ar/cvirtual/cvirteng/cienteng/hteng/htc 0917i/imancia/imancia.htm 2006. (accessed 10/17/2006).*

[60] Grahame-Smith DG. *The Oxford Textbook of Clinical Pharmacology and Drug Therapy*. Oxford: Oxford University Press; 1984.

[61] Maddox DA, Deen WM, Benner BA. Glomerular filtration. In: Windhager EE, editor. Handbook of Physiology, Section 8: *Renal Physiology*, Vol.1. New York, Oxford: American Physiological Society, Oxford University Press; 1992;545-638.

[62] Goodenough DA. Gap junction dynamics and intercellular communication. *Pharmacol Rev*, 1979; 30:383-392.

[63] Sporns O, Seelig FF.Turing structures in an enzyme-induction system with gap junction-mediated non-linear diffusion. *BioSystems*, 1986;19: 237-245.

[64] Geelen G, Latinen T, Hartikainen J, Länsimies E, Bergström K, Niskanen L. Gender influence on vasoactive hormones at rest and during head-up tilt in healthy humans. *J Applied Physiol,* 2002;92: 1401-1408.

[65] Crotty TP. The venous valve agger and plasma noradreneline-mediated venodilator feedback. *Phlebology*, 2007;22(3): 116-130.

[66] Cannon RO, Rosing DR, Maron BJ, Leon MB, Bonow RO, Watson RM et al. Myocardial ischaemia in patients with hypertrophic cardiomyopathy:contribution of inadequate vasodilator reserve and elevated ventricular filling pressure. *Circulation*, 1985;71:234-243..

[67] Crotty TP. Contraction in the smooth muscle cell. *Medical Hypotheses*, 1999:53(5):432-446.

[68] Ludmer PL, Selwyn AP, Shook TL, Wayne RR, Mudge GH, Alexander RW et al. Paradoxical constriction induced by acetycholine in atherosclerotic artery. *NEJM*, 1986;315: 1046-1051.

[69] Vrints CJ, Bult H, Bosmans J, Herman AG, Snoeck JP. Paradoxical vasoconstriction as a result of acetycholine and serotonin in diseased human coronary arteries. *Eur Heart J*, 1992;13: 824-831.

[70] Rodbard S. Flow through collapsible tubes: augmented flow produced by resistance at the outlet. *Circulation*, 1955;11: 280-287.

[71] Rice AJ, Leeson CR, Long JP. Localization of venoconstrictor responses. *J Pharmacol Exp Ther*, 1966;154: 539-54.

[72] Epstein S. Über die Struktur normaler und ektatischer Venen. *Virchows Arch Path Anat,* 1887;108:103-123.

[73] Morgagni GB, Epistola XV. In: Larber A, editor, *Epistola Anatomica II*, Lugduni Batavorum: Cornelius Haak; 1765; 284-315.

[74] Minkov M, Kanellaki-Kyparrissi M, Marinov G, Koliakou K, Knyazhev V, Kovatchev D. Venous valve agger in non-varicose and varicose great saphenous vein: clinico-morphological considerations. *Ann Proc Bulg Med Assoc,* 1989;4: 65-66.

[75] Corcos L, De Anna D, Dini M et al. Proximal long saphenous vein valves in primary venous insufficiency. *J Mal Vasc* (Paris), 2000;25: 27-36.

[76] Vankov VN. Stroenie Ven. Moskva: *Medicina*; 1974.

[77] Crotty TP. An investigation of radial reflux in an isolated peripheral canine vein segment. *Phlebology*, 1995;10: 115-121.

[78] Crotty TP. Increased responsiveness of the canine lateral saphenous vein segment to noradrenaline when flow from its lumen to its network of vasa vasorum was obstructed. *Ir J Med Sci*, 1988;157(11):365.

[79] Silverberg A, Shaha SD, Haymond MW, Cryer PE. Norepinephrine: hormone and transmitter in man. *Am J Physiol*, 1978;234: E252-256.

[80] Crotty TP. Is circulating noradrenaline the cause of varicose veins? *Medical Hypotheses*, 1991;34: 243-251.

[81] Crotty TP. Postenotic dilatation in arteries and the role of turbulence *Medical Hypotheses*, 1994; 42:367-370.

[82] Mäkivaara LA, Ahti TM, Luukkaala T, Hakama M, Laurikka JO. Arterial disease but not hypertension predisposes to varicose veins. *Phlebology*, 2008;23(3):142-146.

[83] Furchgott RF, Zawadski JV. The obligatory role of endothelial cells in relaxation of arterial smooth muscle by acetylcholine. *Nature*, 1980;288: 373-376.

[84] Taylor P. Cholinergic agents. In: Gilman AG, Rall TW, Nies A, Taylor P, editors. *Goodman and Gilman's The Pharmacological Basis of Therapeutics 8th ed.* Oxford: Pergamon Press Oxford; 1990; 122-149.

[85] King ESJ. The genesis of varicose veins. *Aust NZ J Surg*, 1950;20: 126-133.

[86] Browse NL, Burnand KG, Lea Thomas M. editors. *Diseases of the Veins. 1st Ed.* London: Edward Arnold; 1988.

[87] Baron HC, Cessaro S. The role of arteriovenous shunts in the aetiology of varicose veins. *J Vasc Surg*, 1986;4:124-128.

[88] Curri SB. Significato delle alterazioni anatomo funzionali dei vasa venorum nelle pathogenesi del danno parietale venosos e delle malattia varicose. *Flebolinfologio*, 1991;2: 23-42.

[89] Crotty TP. The corrupted feedback hypothesis: a hypothesis on the aetiology of varicose veins. *Medical Hypotheses*, 2003; 61: 605-616.

[90] Tacoenn A, Lebard C, Poullain JC, Gerentes I, Zucarelli F. *Oxygen tension in the wall of varicose and normal veins.* In: Negu SD, Janet G, Coleridge Smith PD editors. Phlebology. Berlin: Springer; 1995; 123-128.

[91] Gowlands Hopkins NF, Spinks TJ, Rhodes CG, Ranicar ASO, Jamieson CW. Positron emission tomography in venous ulceration and liposclerosis: study of regional tissue function. *BMJ*, 1983;286:333-336.

[92] Haardt B. A comparision of the histochermical enzyme pattern in normal and varicose veins. Phlebology, 1987;2:135-158.

[93] Wegmann R, El Sammanoudy FA, Olivier C, Retorri R. Histochemical studies on the wall of varicose veins: the human saphenous vein. *Ann Histochim*,1974;19: 285-292.

[94] Marinov G, Vancov V. Early changes of the smooth muscle cell (SMC) and extracellular matrix in the wall of varicose veins. *Verh Anat* (Jena), 1991; 84 (Anat Anz Suppl 168): 99-100.

[95] Kreysel HW, Nissen HP, Enghofer E. A possible role of lysozymal enzymes in the pathogenesis of varicosis and the reduction in their serum activity by Venostatin. *VASA*, 1983;12: 377-382.

[96] Shields DA, Andaz SK, Sarin S, Scurr JH, Coleridge Smith PD. Plasma elastase in venous disease. Br J Surg, 1994; 81: 1496-1499.

[97] Lassman G, Gottlob R. Die Veränderungen des gefässeigenen Nervensystems bei varizen. *Wien Med Wochenschr*, 1968;118:224-225.

[98] Darke SG. The morphology of recurrent varicose veins. *Eur J Vasc Surg*,1992;6: 512-517.

[99] Geirer A, Meinhardt H. A theory of biological pattern formation. Kybernetick, 1972;12:30-39.

[100] Crank J. *The Mathematics of Diffusion*. Oxford:Clarendon Press:1975.

[101] Utall WR. *The Psychobiology of Sensory Coding*. New York: Harper and Row; 1973.

[102] Von Békésy G. Mach band type lateral inhibition in different sense organs. *J Gen Physiol*, 1967;50: 519-532.

[103] Meinhardt H, Geirer A. Application of a theory of biological pattern formation based on lateral inhibition. *J Cell Sci*, 1974;15:321-346.

[104] *Cellular Aspects of Smooth Muscle Function*. Kao CY, Carsten ME. editors. Cambridge: CambridgeUniversity Press; 1997.

[105] Motta PM, ed. *Ultrastructure of Smooth Muscle*. Kluwer Academic, Boston, 1990.

[106] Kargacin GJ, Cooke PH, Abramson SB, Fay FS. Periodic organization of the contractile apparatus in smooth muscle revealed by the motion of dense bodies in single cell. *J Cell Biol*,1989;108:1465-1475.

[107] Small JV. Structure-function relationships in smooth muscle: the missing link. *BioEssays,* 1995;17:785-792.

[108] Naitoh Y, Eckert R. Ionic mechanisms controlling behavioural responses of Paramecium to mechanical stimulus. *Science*, 1969;164:963-965.

[109] Levitan H, Tauc L. Acetycholine receptors: topographic distribution and pharmacological properties of two receptor types on a single molluscan neurone. *J Physiol* (Lond),1972;222:537-558.

[110] Ratliff F. Mach Bands: Quantitative Studies on Neural Networks in the Retina. San Francisco: *Holden-Day*, 1965.

[111] Kuffler SW. Neurons in the retina: organization, inhibition and excitation. *Cold Spring Harb Symp Quant Biol*, 1952;17:2381-2392.

[112] Kobilka BK. Adrenergic receptor structure and activation. *Pharmacol Communications,* 1995;6:119-124.

[113] Gabella G. General aspects of the fine structure of smooth muscles. In: Motta PM editor. *Ultrastructure of Smooth Muscle*. Boston: Kluwer Academic;1990;1-22.

[114] Murphy RA. What is special about smooth muscle? The significance of crossbridge regulation. *FASEBJ*, 1994;8:311-318.

[115] Sheid CR, Honeyman TW, Fay FS. Mechanism of β-adrenergic relaxation of smooth muscle. *Nature*, 1979;277:32-36.

[116] Scotland R, Vallance P, Ahluwalia A. On the regulation of tone in vasa vasorum. *Cardiovascular Res,* 1999;41:237-45.

[117] Quillen J, Selke F, Banitt P, Harrison D. The effect of norepinephrine on the coronary circulation. *J Vasc Res*, 1992;29:2-7.

[118] Williams JK, Armstrong ML, Heistad DD. Vasa vasorum in atherosclerotic arteries: responses to vasoactive stimuli and regression of atherosclerosis. *Circ Res,* 1988;62:515-523.

[119] Henriksen JK,Ring-Larsen H, Christensen NJ. Hepatic intestinal uptake and release of catecholamines in alcoholic cirrhosis. Evidence of enhanced hepatic intestinal sympathetic nervous activity. *Gut,* 1987;28:1637-1642.

In: Varicose Veins   ISBN 978-1-61209-841-8
Editor: Andrea L. Nelson   © 2011 Nova Science Publishers, Inc.

Chapter 2

THE ROLE OF INFLAMMATION IN THE VARICOSE VEIN PATHOLOGY: NEW INSIGHTS

Lourdes del Rio Solá[1], José Antonio González-Fajardo[1], Mariano Sánchez Crespo[2] and Carmen García-Rodríguez[2]*

[1]Hospital Clinico Universitario de Valladolid, Valladolid, Spain
[2]Instituto de Biologia y Genética Molecular (CSIC-UVA), Valladolid, Spain

ABSTRACT

The pathogenesis of chronic venous disease, a complex and common pathology affecting the lower extremities, is still poorly understood. Accumulating evidence supports the role of inflammation as a mechanism underlying the physiopathology of chronic venous disease. In this review, we will carry out an overview of the role of inflammation in the varicose vein pathology, focusing on recent data that supports the use of pharmacological tools to decrease the production of inflammatory mediators or to block their effects, as a complementary therapeutic approach.

* Correspondence to: Dr. Carmen Garcia-Rodriguez. Instituto de Biologia y Genética Molecular (CSIC-UVA), C/Sanz y Forés 3, laboratory E10 47003. Valladolid, Spain. Phone: +34-983-184841. Fax: +34-983-184800. E-mail: cgarcia@ibgm.uva.es.

The most accepted mechanism linking venous hypertension to the changes in the macro and microcirculation is the leukocyte "trapping" model, according to which leukocytes infiltrate the venous wall and valves and migrate across the postcapillarvenules endothelium, thus leading to wall remodeling and valvular destruction. An incipient inflammatory focus in the vascular intima or media, the activation of endothelial cells by hypoxia, or altered hemodynamics, might cause the leukocytes to leave the circulation. In addition, fluid shear stress can contribute to leukocyte activation, and nitric oxide donors and inflammatory mediators can modulate the response. In the last decade, several reports have shown the involvement of molecules implicated in the inflammatory response such as adhesion molecules and cytokines, especially vascular cellular adhesion molecule-1, transforming growth factor-β, interleukin (IL)-6, IL-8 and matrix metalloproteinases, as well as the transcription factor hypoxia inducible factor-1 α in varicose vein disease. Additionally, in support of the leukocyte "trapping" model, recent data from our group has disclosed a correlation between elevated levels of chemotactic cytokines and varicose veins, specifically monocyte-chemoattractant protein-1, IL-8, interferon-inducible protein-10, RANTES, macrophage-inflammatory protein (MIP)-1α and MIP-1β. Furthermore, recent findings show that acetylsalicylic acid (ASA) treatment of patients with varicose syndrome accelerated healing and delayed recurrence of venous ulceration, suggesting that drugs that diminish leukocyte activation seemed to benefit ulcer healing and could be used as a complementary treatment. In addition to studies with human tissues, several animal model studies have suggested that inhibition of the early stages of inflammation offers potential targets that could be effective for the treatment of venous disease. In summary, recent reports highlight the impact of inflammation and hypoxia on varicose vein pathogenesis, and open the avenue to future preventive and therapeutic designs.

1. INTRODUCTION

Chronic Venous Disease (CVD) is a complex and common pathology affecting the lower limbs and is manifested by a range of different conditions of venous insufficiency including varicose vein and venous ulcers (Eberhardt RT et al 2005; Bergan JJ et al, 2006; 355:488-98; Somers P et al 2006). The severity of all chronic diseases is classified by the CEAP system according to clinical, anatomical, and pathological categories (Eklof B et al, 2009). Positive family history, age, sex,pregnancy, and lifestyle are important risk factors for varicose vein formation. The diversity of signs and symptoms associated with chronic venous disease are thought to be related to venous hypertension, which in most cases is caused by a reflux through incompetent valves, but also by a venous outflow obstruction and failure of the calf-muscle pump (Bergan JJ *et al*, 2006). The venous hypertension is caused to a large degree by weak, worn or damaged valves in the veins of the legs that prevent them from closing properly and allows the blood to flow back entering also smaller veins and accumulating in the leg tissues, therefore leading to oedema. In addition, decreased delivery of oxygen to the leg tissues leads to inflammation and pain. Venous ulceration occurs when valves fail in the deep, superficial, or perforating veins, which leads to impairment of the venous return in the lower extremities.

The pathogenesis of CVD is still poorly understood. Several models have been proposed to explain the causes of the disease, like the fibrin cuff formation that would cause tissue hypoxia, and the growth factor trapping, which are theories that have been disproven over time (reviewed in Pappas PJ *et al*, 2007). The so-called white cell trapping hypothesis (Coleridge-Smith P *et al*, 2003) remains the most accepted mechanism despite its limitations. It is currently thought that during the development of CVD, a sequence of pathophysiological events occur, which include an increase in the endothelial permeability, angiogenesis and microvascular restructuring, as well as circulating cell entrapment and endothelial adhesion, leukocyte activation, tissue proteolytic activity, and valve failure (Schmid-Schönbein G, 2008). In the last decade, considerable progress has been made in understanding the mechanisms that underlie these diverse manifestations, in particular the role of inflammation in the initiation and progression of the disease. In this review, we will give an overview of the role of inflammation reactions in CVD pathology, focusing on the inflammatory mediators associated to the disease, and on recent data providing evidence for the potential use of pharmacological tools for the treatment of CVD (Bergan JJ *et al*, 2006; Sprague A *et al*, 2009; Gohel *et al*, 2010).

2. INFLAMMATION AND CHRONIC VENOUS DISEASE

Inflammation is a tissue repair mechanism that is activated in response to damage and that terminates when the injurious stimulus is removed; however, under certain conditions the repair and healing processes do not achieve resolution, leading to a chronic inflammatory state and disease, i.e., CVD (Schmid-Schonbein GW, 2008). Growing evidence from both humans and experimental models has highlighted the role of inflammation in the pathogenesis of CVD. Its participation in the initiation and progression of venous disease is increasingly accepted, and it is clear that all clinical stages of CVD result in systemic inflammatory response (Schmid-Schönbein G, 2008). In fact, signs of an inflammatory response are already detectable at the early stages of CVD and may be involved in the development of primary venous valve dysfunction (reviewed in Schmid-Schonbein GW, 2008). Among the early microvascular manifestations of inflammation is the elevated endothelial permeability, a process that involves the opening of interendothelial junctions (Schmid-Schönbein G, 2007). In addition, it has been reported that valves in veins from CVD patients show clear signs of inflammation, which include activated endothelium (Takase S *et al*, 2000), leukocyte adhesion to the endothelium and migration into the valve leaflets and venous wall (Takase S *et al*, 1999), and immune cell infiltration, i.e., T lymphocytes and monocytes (Ono T *et al*, 1998). Moreover, varicose veins from patients with a family history of CVD showed elevated levels of mast cell infiltration, therefore suggesting that inflammation may be a cause rather than a consequence of CVD (Kakkos SK *et al*, 2003). Furthermore, several animal models of venous hypertension have also highlighted the crucial role of inflammation in the CVD, and those studies suggest that early stages of the inflammatory cascade are potential targets for therapeutic intervention (reviewed in Bergan JJ *et al*, 2008).

The factors triggering inflammation in the CVD are still unknown, although current evidence suggests possible mechanisms including hypoxia, humoral stimulation, fluid shear stress changes and endothelial distension under the influence of elevated venous pressure (Schmid-Schönbein G, 2008). Inflammation is a process susceptible to be manipulated; therefore knowing the mechanisms that cause inflammation and prevent its resolution will be useful not only to understand the pathogenesis of the disease, but also to develop new therapeutic approaches for prevention and treatment.

The machinery of inflammation comprises not only a cellular component, which includes circulating immune and vascular cells, but also a molecular component, which includes structural molecules from the extracellular matrix as well as soluble inflammatory mediators. We will focus on the main cells involved in the inflammation underlying CVD, as well as the inflammatory mediators that have been associated with the disease.

2.1. Types and Distribution of Cells

2.1.1. Leukocytes

The most accepted mechanism linking venous hypertension to the changes in the macro and microcirculation is the white cell trapping hypothesis. In fact, leukocyte infiltration into the venous leaflets is one of the hallmarks of the inflammatory process. The first evidence of abnormal leukocyte activity in the pathophysiology of CVD came from the description of leukocyte blood depletion after venous stasis, suggesting that leukocyte might be trapped in the microcirculation (Thomas PR *et al*, 1988). Based on these and other data from the literature, it was hypothesized that white cells become trapped in the venous microcirculation secondary to venous hypertension and subsequently slow the blood flow, which in turn leads to hypoxia and leukocyte activation that can release toxic metabolites, therefore causing damage to the micro-circulation and the overlying skin (Coleridge-Smith PD *et al*, 1988). Support for the leukocyte-trapping model comes from immunohistological and ultrastructural studies that have revealed the existence of leukocytes adhering and transmigrating into the venous wall (Takase S *et al*, 1999; Ono T *et al*, 1998), and in the skin from CVD patients (Pappas PJ *et al*, 1997), and from studies demonstrating inappropriate leukocyte activation in venous disease (Saharay M *et al*, 1997). Many other studies have reported evidence for the leukocyte-trapping model (Coleridge-Smith PD, 2003).

There is significant evidence that increased leukocyte adhesion and activation have been reported to be associated with venous disease (Coleridge *et al*, 2003; Boisseau MR, 2007). Under conditions of high venous pressure, leukocytes are trapped in the microcirculation of the lower limbs (Thomas PR *et al*, 1988) due to their stiff cytoplasmic properties and their capacity to express membrane adhesion molecules. In addition, leukocytes may be stimulated in the circulation by mechanisms external to the venous network of the lower extremities. It has been reported that circulating leukocytes in CVD patients are in an altered state of activation and therefore may be involved in leukocyte-mediated injury. Interestingly, patients with chronic venous stasis ulcers had a decreased expression of T lymphocytes markers (Pappas PJ *et al*, 1997), suggesting a decreased capacity for mononuclear cell proliferation in response to various challenges that could explain the clinical observation of poor and prolonged wound healing (Pappas PJ *et al*, 2007).

The types of leukocytes involved in CVD are mostly macrophages and T lymphocytes, and to a much lower extent neutrophils and B lymphocytes. T lymphocytes and macrophages were predominantly observed perivasculary and in the epidermis. A quantitative morphometric assessment of the dermal microcirculation using electron microscopy reported that macrophages and mast cells were the predominant cells observed in patients with CVD dermal skin changes (Pappas *et al,* 1997). This is the same pattern as observed in both acute and chronic experimental rat models of venous hypertension, with elevated levels of tissue leukocytes in skin samples from affected limbs (reviewed in Bergan JJ *et al*, 2008).

The molecular mechanism involved in leukocyte adhesion and activation in CVD patients are beginning to be understood. The evidence in CVD suggests that leukocytes respond to changes in fluid shear stress, although their response differs from that of endothelial cells, and the effect is further amplified by the presence of inflammatory mediators. It is known that blood stasis, which implies lower shear stress, can activate leukocytes and promote their transendothelial migration by means of stimulating the projection of pseudopodia and lamellipodia as well as facilitating adhesion to the endothelium (Coleridge-Smith P *et al*, 2003). At the microvascular level, there might be some differences in white-cell trapping. While leukocyte entrapment in the capillaries might not require membrane adhesion, attachment of leukocytes to postcapillary venules requires adhesion to endothelium via adhesion molecules. In the skin microcirculation, alternative leukocytes become entrapped by adhesion to the endothelium, which is activated by a local process. In fact, it is well accepted that leukocyte adhesion to the membrane of the endothelium of small vessels, especially capillaries and postcapillary venules, play a crucial role on the pathogenesis of CVD (Nicolaides AN, 2005), and several venoactive drugs currently used to treat the disease have beneficial effects by decreasing leukocyte-endothelium adhesion (Gohel MS *et al*, 2009). Interestingly, in addition to having local factors related to venous hypertension, patients with CVD tend to have a systemic increase in leukocyte adhesion. Upon activation, leukocytes secrete inflammatory mediators that induce a cascade of events in which macrophages and fibroblasts are recruited to wound healing sites and stimulated to produce fibroblast mitogens and connective tissue proteins, respectively, thus provoking skin changes in CVD. In fact, degranulation of the leukocytes with an increase of neutrophil elastase and lactoferrin, markers of neutrophils activation, occurs in patients under transient conditions of venous hypertension and with CVD (Boisseau M, 2007). Furthermore, leukocyte infiltration into the venous parenchyma is accompanied by the remodeling of the extracellular matrix, a process that is ultimately responsible for the destruction of the venous valves, and it has been speculated that mast cells and macrophages might function to regulate tissue remodelling, which ultimately causes dermal fibrosis (Coleridge-Smith P *et al*, 2003; Schmid-Schonbein G *et al*, 2001).

2.1.2. Endothelial Cells

Under physiological conditions, the endothelium keeps a vasodilator, antithrombotic, and anti-inflammatory state. However, endothelial cell injury due to an increase in vein wall tension may induce structural changes in the vein wall, and triggers leukocyte infiltration and inflammation, which in turn promote further vein wall damage. When endothelial cells become dysfunctional by the opening of endothelial tight junctions and cell pore formation, there is a subsequent increase of endothelial permeability, one of the early manifestations of CVD. Opening of endothelial junctions is thought to be responsible for macromolecule extravasation and oedema formation, although alternative mechanisms could explain tissue oedema like, i.e., increased transendothelial vesicle transport, formation of transendothelial channels, and alterations in the glycocalyx lining the junctional cleft (Pappas PJ et al, 1997; Saharay M et al, 1998). There are several mediators that can increase the endothelial permeability, including complement protein, platelet activating factor, cytokines, and growth factors (Schmid-Schonbein GW, 2008). It is thought that reduction of endothelial permeability may be a useful therapeutic target for early intervention, since it may interrupt the inflammatory cascade at one of its earlier steps (Bergan JJ et al, 2006).

As mentioned earlier, another important step in the development of CVD is the increased adhesion of inflammatory cells to the endothelium. Activation of the endothelium is known to stimulate the increase of adhesion molecules on the membrane, thus increasing the leukocyte adhesion to endothelium characteristic of CVD. In addition, endothelial cell activation stimulates the release of growth factors, thus leading to smooth muscle cell proliferation and migration (Bergan JJ et al, 2006; Lim CS et al, 2011a).

2.1.3. Other Cells

Other vascular cells like smooth muscle cells and dermal fibroblasts could be functionally altered during the CVD (Raffetto JD, 2007). Dermal fibroblast from CVD patients showed reduction of the proliferation rate and motility, as well as diminished regulation by growth factors (Raffetto JD, 2007). During the development of CVD, smooth muscle cells respond to injury or medial hypoxia, by synthesizing extracellular matrix molecules and protease inhibitors that promote remodeling. However, it is thought that these cell rearrangements are not primary factors for CVD, but secondary to changes due to a compensatory age mechanism for an increase of volume pressure of the lower extremities (Somers P et al, 2006).

2.2. Extracelular Matrix

The extracellular matrix is a three-dimensional structure essential for the functionality of vessel walls that is composed of several molecules like elastin, collagens, proteoglycans, and structural glycoproteins. It is known that in response to injury, i.e., lipid deposition, hypoxia, enzyme secretion, and reactive oxygen species, the extracellular matrix molecules are hydrolyzed by proteases like matrix metalloproteinases (MMPs) and leukocyte elastase. During the development of the CVD, migrated leukocytes localize around capillaries and postcapillary venules, and the perivasculary space is surrounded by extracellular matrix proteins that form a perivascular cuff, erroneously referred to as the fibrin cuff, which it is thought to be built to maintain vascular architecture in response to increased mechanical load (Pappas PJ, 2007). Immunohistochemical studies have shown that the perivasculary cuff is a ring of extracellular matrix proteins consisting of collagen types I and III, fibronectin, vitronectin, laminin, tenascin, and fibrin. In patients with CVD, the proportion of collagen type III is significantly decreased in cultured smooth muscle cells and dermal fibroblast, indicating a deficiency in collagen type III (Sansilvestri-Morel P *et al*, 2003). Much evidence suggests that the remodeling of the extracellular matrix is due to activation of several MMPs. Interestingly, recent evidence suggests that changes in the vein wall may even precede valvular incompetence and reflux, which have been considered for a long time the primary cause of varicose veins (Lim CS *et al*, 2011a). In pathological conditions like CVD, the balance between proteases and their inhibitors is temporally destroyed through the induction of MMPs or the secretion of enzymes by inflammatory cells (Jacob MP *et al*, 2001). Smooth muscle cells have the capacity to respond to injury through the synthesis of extracellular matrix molecules and protease inhibitors, however, the newly synthesized extracellular matrix is never functionally optimal. Therefore, any therapeutic manipulation aimed to regulate vein wall remodeling by altering the protease/inhibitor balance must be perfectly controlled, because an accumulation of abnormal extracellular matrix may have unexpected adverse effects.

2.3. Inflammatory Mediators

At the molecular level, increasing experimental and clinical evidence has shown the involvement of inflammatory molecules in the varicose vein disease (Table I). The interest of these studies resides in the fact that inflammatory mediators could be used as diagnosis tools as well as therapeutically relevant targets for the design of new pharmacological treatments for the CVD.

Table I. Inflammatory mediators that have been associated with CVD

INFLAMMATORY MEDIATORS INVOLVED IN CVD	(References)
Adhesion molecules: *ICAM-1, VCAM-1, E-selectin, ELAM-1*	Saharay M, 1998 Satokawa H, 2002
Metalloproteinases: *MMP-1 , -2, -3,- 7, and -9* *TIMP-1, TIMP-3*	Badier-Commander C, 2000 Aravind B, 2010
Cytokines: *TNF* *IL6* *Chemokines like MCP-1, MIP1α, MIP-1β, IL-8, IP-10, RANTES*	Takase S, 2000 Murphy MA, 2002 Del Rio Solá ML ,2009
Growth factors: *TGF-β1 and TGF-β1 receptor II* *VEGF* *PDGF*	Pappas PJ, 1999; Kowalwesky R, 2010 Shoab SS, 1998; Howlader MH, 2004 Margolis DJ, 2009
Hypoxia inducible factors: *HIF-1α, -2α*	Ghaderian SM, 2010; Lim CS, 2011b
Oxidative stress: *Elastase* *Superoxide dismutase, malondialdehyde, nitric oxide*	Shields DA, 1994 Karatepe O, 2010
Lipid mediators: *Eicosanoids like TXA$_2$ and prostacyclin* *Lyso-PC, PC and sphyngomyelin*	Haynes DF, 1990 Tanaka H, 2010

2.3.1. Adhesion Molecules

It has been reported that several molecules involved in the leukocyte-endothelium adhesion process might play a role in CVD pathogenesis; among these molecules are membrane adhesion molecules expressed in circulating leukocytes and vascular endothelial cells, i.e. vascular-cell adhesion molecule (VCAM)-1, intercellular adhesion molecule (ICAM)-1, E-selectin, CD11b, etc. The first step in the process of leukocyte-endothelium adhesion is the rolling of circulating leukocytes along the endothelial surface, a slow motion stage that requires the transient binding of L-selectin on the leukocyte surface to E-selectin on endothelial cells (Yong K *et al*, 1990). The next step is firm adhesion of leukocytes that requires the expression of members of the integrin family, including CD18/CD11b (MAC-1, $\alpha_M\beta_2$), which binds to the adhesion molecule ICAM-1 therefore promoting leukocyte-endothelium interaction, a process that precedes the migration out of the vasculature and degranulation.

In patients with CVD, the induction of venous hypertension by standing for 30 minutes diminishes the levels of L-selectin and the integrin CD11b on circulating neutrophils and monocytes, reflecting their trapping in the microcirculation, while plasma levels of soluble L-selectin increased, reflecting the shedding of these molecules from leukocyte surfaces during leukocyte-endothelium adhesion (Saharay M *et al*, 1997). Several studies have shown high levels of adhesion molecules in varicose veins (reviewed in Ghaderian SM *et al*, 2010). Initial studies showed that basal plasma levels of ICAM-1, endothelial leukocyte adhesion molecule-1, and VCAM-1 were higher in patients with CVD than in control subjects, and further increased in response to venous stasis. Moreover, the levels of soluble ICAM-1 and E-selectin were significantly elevated in the serum of patients with CVD (Saharay M *et al*, 1998), which may reflect endothelial damage in response to venous hypertension.

Furthermore, a comparative study between competent and incompetent valves from patients with primary varicose veins revealed a higher expression of adhesion molecules at the venous wall of incompetent valves when compared with competent valves (Satokawa H *et al*, 2002).

2.3.2. MMPs

During the development of CVD, weakening of the vein wall due to extracellular matrix degradation and remodeling occurs and it might contribute to the destruction of venous valves. Histological and ultrastructural studies of varicose veins have found structural changes in the vein wall characterized by an increase in the collagen content and rearrangement of elastin fibers

(Woodside KJ *et al*, 2003). Tissue remodeling and matrix deposition are processes controlled by MMPs and tissue inhibitors of MMPs (TIMPs). MMPs are a family of proteolytic enzymes such as collagenase, gelatinase, and stromelysines with the capacity to degrade several components of the extracellular matrix, and known to be involved in the extracellular remodeling occurring in CVD (reviewed in Raffetto JD *et al*, 2008). It has been reported that MMP-1, MMP-2, MMP-3, MMP-7 and MMP-9, and TIMP-1 and TIMP-3 are upregulated in varicose veins (Raffetto JD *et al*, 2008). Moreover, chronic dermal ulcers are characterized by excessive proteolytic activity, the MMPs levels in wound fluid from chronic wounds are higher than from acute wounds, and healing is associated with reduced MMP activity (reviewed in Raffetto JD *et al*, 2008).

In general, MMPs and TIMPs are not constitutively expressed, but are induced temporally in response to exogenous signals such as various proteases, cytokines or growth factors, cell-matrix interactions and altered cell-cell interactions. Among these signals, urokinase plasminogen activators may activate MMP-2. In addition, it has been shown that MMP-2-induced venous dilation through the activation of K+ channel and hyperpolarization might be relevant to varicose vein formation (Raffetto JD *et al,* 2007). Interestingly, changes in MMP and TIMP production may similarly modulate the tissue fibrosis of the lower extremity in CVD patients. Several studies have shown increased levels of MMP-2 and 9 as well as TIMP-1, in the exudates of patients with venous ulcers compared to acute wounds, thus suggesting that active tissue remodeling is occurring in patients with CVD (Raffetto JD *et al* 2008). In addition, it has been reported that the production of collagen and TIMP is regulated by prolonged and continuous production of transforming growth factor (TGF)-β_1, a growth factor known to cause fibrosis. The elevated level of active TGF-β1 in the dermis of CVD patients suggests a regulatory role for TGF-β_1 in the synthesis and activity of MMP and TIMP (Badier-Commander C *et al*, 2000). Interestingly, an imbalance of the TIMP/MMP ratio in varicose veins has been proposed as a possible explanation for the extracellular matrix accumulation associated with CVD (Badier-Commander C *et al*, 2000; Bujan J *et al*, 2000). Moreover, a recent study has linked morphological changes in varicose vein walls with MMP/TIMP balance and demonstrated that an increase of TIMP expression favors deposition of connective tissue and thus thicker vein wall, by a mechanism that reduces matrix turnover by abrogation of protease activity (Aravind B *et al*, 2010).

Overexpression of other proteins from the extracellular matrix like the matrix Gla protein have been reported to contribute to venous wall remodeling by affecting proliferation and mineralization processes probably through impaired carboxylation (Cario-Toumaniantz C *et al*, 2007). Further studies are required to elucidate the specific roles in the pathogenesis of CVD of other extracellular matrix components that have been associated to remodeling and are overexpressed in human varicose veins, i.e. collagen III, dermatopontin, and tenascin C (Cario-Toumaniantz C *et al*, 2007).

2.3.3. Cytokines

Cytokines are polypeptides with a wide range of effects. Several cytokines have been associated to CVD, including tumor necrosis (TNF)-α, granulocyte/monocyte colony stimulating factor (GM-CSF), interleukin (IL)-6, and chemokines (Gohel *et al*, 2008). It is well accepted that cytokines are part of the inflammatory response underlying CVD (Takase S *et al*, 2000) and recent studies support this idea (Gohel MS *et al*, 2008). However, their exact role on CVD remains to be elucidated. The use of periulcer injection of GM-CSF for the treatment of venous ulcers leads to mixed results (reviewed in O'Donnell TF *et al*, 2006). Epidemiological studies have found the association of elevated levels of cytokines with increased vascular risk (Sprague A *et al*, 2009). In addition, inflammatory cytokines may be involved in vein valve insufficiency (Takase S *et al*, 2000). It has been reported that venous stasis causes the activation of monocyte/macrophages and the release of cytokines (Takase S *et al*, 2000; Satokawa H *et al*, 2002). Moreover, non-healing wounds have been shown to express higher concentrations of pro-inflammatory cytokines, such as TNF-α and IL-1 than healing wounds (Murphy MA *et al*, 2002), and compression therapy diminishes levels of cytokines such as GM-CSF, IL1-α, IL1-β, IFN-γ, and IL12p40 in ulcer tissue (Beidler SK *et al*, 2009). Furthermore, a recent pilot study has shown the presence of increased levels of TNF-α within recalcitrant venous leg ulcers (Charles CA *et al*, 2009). Interestingly, it is thought that plasma levels of pro-inflammatory cytokines like TNF-α and IL-6 may be used as early markers for varicose veins (Sprague A *et al*, 2009).

Chemokines are small molecular weight cytokines with the capacity to recruit immune cells. In support of the leukocyte "trapping" model, recent data from our group has disclosed a correlation between elevated levels of chemotactic cytokines and varicose veins, specifically monocyte-chemoattractant protein (MCP)-1, IL-8, interferon-inducible protein-10, RANTES, macrophage-inflammatory protein (MIP)-1α, and MIP-1β (Del Rio Sola ML *et al*, 2009). Interestingly, these chemokines can recruit many cells to the varicose vein wall, thus contributing to amplify and perpetuate the inflammatory response. Furthermore, recent findings show that acetylsalicylic acid (ASA) treatment of patients with varicose syndrome accelerated healing and delayed recurrence of venous ulceration (Del Río Solá ML *et al*, in press), suggesting that drugs with the capacity of diminishing leukocyte activation could be used as complementary treatment.

2.3.4. Growth Factors

Microscopic studies reveal that the proliferation of vessels characteristic of lipodermatosclerotic skin is mostly due to increased elongation and tortuosity of vessels. Vascular endothelial growth factor (VEGF), known to be increased in plasma from patients with CVD (Shoab SS *et al*, 1998; Howlader MH *et al*, 2004), might be a candidate for promoting changes in the skin capillaries, which become elongated and tortuous and may take on a glomerular appearance in lipodermatosclerosis. In addition, VEGF is known to induce the expression of adhesion molecules, its expression is desregulated under changes of blood shear stress and the inflammatory conditions, and the level of VEGF increases with the severity of the disease (reviewed in Pappas PJ *et al*, 2007; Schmid-Schönbein G, 2007). Another feature of lipodermatero-sclerosis is fibrosis of the skin. Studies with TGF-β_1, an important inductor of fibrosis, revealed that this growth factor could stimulate the production of collagen by dermal fibroblast, thus contributing to dermal fibrosis (Pappas PJ *et al*, 1999). In addition, elevated levels of TGF-β_1 and fibroblast growth factor (FGF)-β have been found in the walls of varicose veins (Badier-Commander *et al*, 2001). Immunohistochemical analyses have demonstrated the expression of TGF-β1 and macroglobulin in the interstitium of perivascular cuffs, thus indicating that these molecules are distributed abnormally in the dermis and may contribute to tissue remodeling and fibrosis. Interestingly, recent evidence has shown that TGF-β_1 levels in wound fluid mirrored ulcer healing in a study population, although individual variations in cytokine concentration in the wound and serum will limit their value as markers (Gohel MS *et al*, 2008). Moreover, a recent article suggests the involvement of the TGF-β_1 receptor II in extracellular matrix remodeling related to TGF-β_1 and supports its role in the disease pathogenesis (Kowalewski R *et al*, 2010). Furthermore, a recent report also suggests that the failure of exogenous TGF-β_1 to accelerate healing in chronic wounds can be explained by attenuation of the TGF-β_1 signaling observed in chronic venous ulcers (Pastar I *et al*, 2010).

The involvement of other growth factors such as platelet-derived growth factor (PDGF), has also been investigated in CVD patients. In fact, a phase I study has been performed to test the initial safety, feasibility, and biologic plausibility of using an adenoviral construct expressing PDGF-β to treat venous leg ulcer disease (Margolis DJ et al, 2009).

2.3.5. Hypoxia-Inducible Factors (HIF)

The evidence for hypoxia as a causal factor in varicosities has remained inconclusive, mainly due to heterogeneity and poor design of in vivo studies..Recent evidence has highlighted the role of hypoxia in the pathogenesis of CVD (Ghaderian SM et al, 2010; Lim CS et al, 2011a). It was known that an abnormality of oxygen delivery to vascular tissue leads to changes in the vein wall, such as endothelial damage and smooth muscle proliferation, therefore suggesting that inflammatory changes observed in varicose veins are due to hypoxic damage to the endothelial cells (Michiels C et al, 2000). Recent molecular studies in a rat model have shown that hypoxia was able to cause inflammatory changes and vein wall remodeling similar to those observed in varicosities (Lim CS et al, 2011b). Based on these observations, the authors proposed a mechanism in which prolonged mechanical stretch is associated with the induction of some nuclear transcriptional factor that regulate genes involved in oxygen homeostasis, HIFs, that cause an increase of MMP expression, which in turn leads to venous dilation and further venous pressure increase (Lim SJ et al, 2011). In addition, a recent report shows the expression of HIF-1α in varicose vein specimens but not in control saphenous veins, and that the alterations of the intima in varicose veins might be influenced by hypoxia (Ghaderian SM et al, 2010). Further studies are needed to improve our understanding of the role of hypoxia in the pathogenesis of the CVD, and to identify potential therapeutic targets for the disease.

2.3.6. Oxidative Stress

Oxidative stress is an important pathophysiologic mechanism in the progression of several diseases, including CVD. A higher oxidative stress in the valvular tissue may contribute to CVD, since increased neutrophil degranulation is observed in patients with venous disease (Shields DA et al, 1994). It has been hypothesized that leukocyte infiltration into valve leaflets and subsequent degranulation and release of toxic metabolites might contribute to the enzymatic degradation of the valve leaflets and venous wall (reviewed in Coleridge-Smith P et al, 2003). In addition, the extravasation of red blood cells leads to oxidative stress as well as elevated ferritin and ferric iron levels in affected skin, and it has been proposed that this could cause the formation of hydroxyl radical formation, potential MMP activation, and development of a local microenvironment that exacerbates tissue damage and delays healing (Wilms H *et al*, 2000). Moreover, recent studies have emphasized the impact of oxidative stress in valvular tissues in patients with CVD at different stages of the disease along with MMPs increases, since superoxide dismutase, malondialdehyde and nitric oxide levels are increased in valve tissue from patients with healing venous ulcer when compared to patients without ulcers (Karatepe O *et al*, 2010).

2.3.7. Lipid Mediators

Hyperlipidemia has been reported in many of the patients with CVD (Evans CJ *et al* 1999). The increase of production of eicosanoids like prostacyclin and thromboxane (TX)-A_2 has been detected in human varicose veins (Haynes DF *et al*, 1990). Recent evidence revealed that even though the serum lipid parameters were similar in patients with varicose and non-varicose veins, an accumulation of lipid mediators, such as lyso-phosphatidylcholine (PC), PC and sphyngomielin, were found around the damaged valvular area in varicose veins (Tanaka H *et al*, 2010). Although further studies are required to understand the initiating mechanism of lipid accumulation, these interesting datas suggest that tissue inflammation associated to abnormal lipid metabolism might contribute to the pathogenesis of the disease (Tanaka H *et al*, 2010).

2.4. Mechanisms for Cell Activation and Inflammation

Several primary mechanisms may stimulate inflammatory cascades in the circulation (Schmid-Schönbein G, 2007) that can be classified into several general categories:

- Positive feedback mechanism: Inflammatory responses are mediated by direct action of plasma inflammatory mediators and may in part be triggered by trauma or by bacterial, viral, or fungal sources (Yamakawa Y et al, 2000). The list of inflammatory mediators is long and include cytokines, MMPs, and growth factors (Gohel MS et al, 2008; Raffetto JD et al, 2008).
- Negative feedback mechanism: This mechanism is based on reduction of anti-inflammatory mediators like nitric oxide, adenosine, glucocorticoids, and anti-inflammatory cytokines.
- Cell-cell interaction and activation: This mechanism involves membrane contact in the form of juxtacrine activation; it occurs

during processes of cell-cell interactions, like endothelial cells and leukocyte adhesion, which subsequently promotes the activation of both cell types (Zimmerman GA et al, 1996).

- Activation by mechanotransduction: This mechanism involves changes in the magnitude and direction of fluid shear stress, which promotes changes on the vascular endothelium (Boisseau M, 2003). Fluid shear stress is a tangential force produced by moving blood acting on the endothelial surface and a function of the velocity gradient of blood near the endothelial surface and the blood viscosity. In fact, modifications in the blood flow field in venules may act as a pro-inflammatory stimulus, since it has been described that low levels of fluid shear stress can lead to leukocyte activation (Fukuda S et al, 2000), through several G-protein coupled receptors that serve as mechanosensors of fluid stress (Makino A et al, 2006).

- Activation by physical transients: Changes in gas concentration like oxygen can promote cell activation and inflammation. As mentioned earlier, hypoxia initiates a cascade of actions that lead to endothelial cell damage, which in turn contributes to CVD pathogenesis (Michiels C et al, 2000; Ghaderian SM et al, 2010).

- Activation by hormonal pathways: The higher incidence of varicose veins in women compared with men suggests the potential role of endogenous sex hormones, and candidates are progesterone, insulin, and others (Miller AP et al, 2004). In women, the action of progesterone may play an important role by reduction of smooth muscle tone, allowing venous distension that could compromise venous valve function (Perrot-Applanat et al, 1995). More recently, the involvement of estrogen receptors α and β in the venous relaxation pathways that lead to venous dilation has been demonstrated in a rat model (Rafetto JD et al, 2010). Although gender differences need to be confirmed in human veins, a recent article supports the notion of a possible causal relationship between sex steroids and varicose veins in males (Kendler M et al, 2010).

- Genetic mechanism: Genetic risk factors are thought to play an important role in the pathogenesis of CVD, although there is some controversy about its real contribution (Fiebig A et al, 2010; Ahti TM et al, 2009). Genetic linkage analysis has revealed the existence of patients with familial risk factors; an imbalance between collagen I and collagen III has been found in proximal segments of human varicose saphenous veins in addition to fragmentation of elastin fibrils (Sansilvestri-Morel P et al, 2001).

During the long-lasting clinical course of CVD, it is likely that several of these mechanisms may contribute to initiate and perpetuate inflammation characteristic of CVD (Schmid-Schönbein G, 2007). Currently, it is thought that crucial mechanisms involved in the development of the CVD include altered fluid shear stress that leads to valve leaflet destruction, and vein wall distension caused by elevation of venous pressure and by tissue remodeling promoted by MMPs that are activated by leukocyte adhesion, hormones, and genetic mechanisms (Schmid-Schönbein G, 2008). The identification of the prevailing mechanism might help to design therapeutic strategies for the treatment of the disease.

3. THERAPEUTICAL APPROACHES TO CVD

Different methods of treatment for CVD are currently available producing short-term efficacy in most cases. However, often it is followed by a high recurrence rate after years. Treatment to block inflammation could be potentially useful to prevent disease-related complications. In fact, several of the presently available drugs attenuate various components of the inflammatory response, particularly the leukocyte-endothelium interaction.

3.1. Current Therapies

3.1.2. Compressive Therapy
The most common therapy is the conservative treatment, which includes compression, exercise, and intermittent elevation (Deatrick K et al, 2010). The compression therapy is performed with graded compression stockings that squeeze the legs, preventing excess blood from flowing backwards, thus leading to hemodynamic benefits. Its exact mechanism of therapy is unknown, although it has been reported that treatment of CVD patients by compression bandage has a distinct anti-inflammatory effect (Junger M et al, 2000), and that a reduction in serum cytokine levels parallels healing of venous ulcers (Murphy MA et al, 2002; Beidler SK et al, 2009). Despite the effectiveness of this therapy in healing and preventing recurrences of ulceration obtained in

several trials, the limitation of this therapy is patience, compliance, and high recurrence rates in some cases (Deatrick K *et al*, 2010).

3.1.3. Surgical And Interventional Treatment

Conventional surgical techniques are commonly used, including ligation and stripping of the saphenous vein, and subfascial endoscopic perforation surgery. Currently, new interventional endovenous treatments have been developed as an alternative to conventional surgery for definitive treatment of varicose syndrome. These therapies include the endovenous laser ablation (EVLA), radio frequency ablation (RFA), and foam sclerotherapy (FS), which have some advantages and disadvantages in comparison with conventional surgery, but the overall symptoms relief rate seems to be comparable (Deatrick K *et al*, 2010). Large and well-conducted randomized trials are still needed to further assess the benefit of these new surgical approaches (Gloviczki P *et al*, 2009).

3.2. Pharmacological Therapy

According to the leukocyte activation model, drugs with anti-inflammatory properties may be beneficial for the treatment of CVD. Several groups of drugs with venoactive properties and some anti-inflammatory properties have been used for its treatment, i.e., coumarins, flavonoids, saponosides and other plant extracts (Eberhardt RT *et al*, 2005). In addition, a number of drugs that modify leukocyte activation have been evaluated in patients with venous ulceration with interesting results (Gohel MS *et al*, 2009; Gohel MS *et al*, 2010). Here we summarize some pharmacological tools in use as well as other potential drugs, the mechanism of action of which is based on targeting inflammatory cascades and mediators.

Table II includes un updated list of the current therapies used in the clinic, as well as novel therapies that could potentially be used as complementary therapies for the treatment of CVD.

Table II. Therapeutic agents for the treatment of CVD

PHARMACOLOGICAL AGENTS	(References)
VENOACTIVE DRUGS:	
Flavonoids	Guilhou JJ, 1997
Hydroxyrutosides	BalmerA , 1980; Pulvertaft TB, 1983; De Jongste AB, 1989; Nocker W, 1990
Other natural drugs (e.g. coumarin, escin etc)	Schmeck-Lindenau HJ, 2003
NON VENOACTIVE DRUGS:	
Prostaglandin E1	Beitner H, 1980; Rudofsky G, 1989
Prostacyclin analogues	Muller B, 1988; Musial J, 1986; Belch JJF, 1987; Werner-Schlenzka H, 1994
Pentoxifylline	Sullivan GW, 1988; Angelides NS, 1989; Colgan MP, 1990; Dale JJ, 1999
Acetylsalicylic acid (ASA)	Layton A, 1994; Ibbotson SH, 1995; Del Río-Solá L, *in press*
Thymosin beta 4 (Tβ4)	Guarnera G, 2010
Calcium dobesilate	Martinez-Zapata MJ, 2008
OTHER POTENTIAL AGENTS:	
HIF inhibitors (e.g. echinomycin, U0126)	Lim CS, 2011b
MMP modulators (e.g. doxocyclin, Ro-28-2653)	Raffetto JD, 2008
Growth factor modulators *(VEGF, TGFβ-1, PDGF)*	Howlader MH, 2004; Pastar I, 2010; Margolis DJ, 2009
Chemokine antagonists	Del Río-Solá ML, 2009

3.2.1. Venoactive Drugs

Venoactive drugs, also called venotonics, vasoprotectors, phlebotonics, phlebotropics, venotropics, and oedema-protective agents, may be of synthetic or plant origin; and are widely used in Europe to relieve venous symptoms in all stages of CVD. It is thought that venotonics have many beneficial effects including repairs of the vein wall, increase of the venous tone, decrease of capillary permeability, improvement of the capillary-venular flow, protection of the connective tissue surrounding the vessels, reduction of protein extravasation, improvement of venous oxygenation, and anti-oxidant action (reviewed in Gohel MS et al, 2010). Venoactive drugs are used either alone or in combination with compressive therapy, and are an alternative to compressive therapy in contraindications such as arterial disorders, skin infections, and intolerance or low patient compliance to compressive stockings.

3.2.1.1. Flavonoids and its Derivatives

The most studied vasoactive agent is a micronized purified flavonoid fraction (MPFF) or Daflon®. The precise mechanism of these γ-benzopyrones is unknown, although it is thought that flavonoids might affect the endothelium and leukocytes by decreasing leukocyte activation and adhesion, by inhibiting inflammatory pathways, and by reducing oedema (Eberhardt RT et al, 2008; Gohel MS et al, 2010). The beneficial effects of this drug on venous leg ulcer healing have been confirmed in a double-blind randomized study (Guilhou JJ et al, 1999). In addition, treatment with MPFF reduces substantially the expression of adhesion molecules like VCAM-1 and ICAM-1, thus suggesting that it might interfere with the leukocyte-endothelium adhesion, and that endothelial damage can be alleviated by the treatment (Coleridge-Smith PD et al, 1997). Moreover, MPFF was effective at inhibiting inflammation induced by venous hypertension in animal models (Takase S et al, 2004). More recently, evidence from a rat model of venous hypertension supports the hypothesis that Daflon® is blocking an early inflammatory signal (Pascarella L et al, 2008). Even though the exact mechanism remains to be identified, this data suggest that blocking the vein wall remodeling of venous valves in venous insufficiency may provide an earlier stage of therapeutic intervention (Pascarella L et al, 2008).

Oxerutins and rutosides are flavonoid derivatives used in the management of the symptoms of venous diseases,which have the ability to decrease capillary permeability and free radicals (reviewed in Pappas PJ et al, 2007; Gohel MS et al, 2010). Their effects have been evaluated in numerous randomized studies that consistently showed improvement of symptoms associated with CVD, i.e. reducing aching, tiredness, swelling, muscle cramps, and oedema (Balmer A *et al*, 1980; Pulvertaft TB *et al*, 1983; De Jongste AB *et al*, 1989; Nocker W *et al*, 1990). However, these drugs do not have any effect on preventing venous leg ulcer healing and recurrence, therefore suggesting that oedema might not be an important process in the development of leg ulceration.

3.2.1.2. Other Natural Venoactive Drugs

Saponosides like horse chesnut extracts (also called escin) have been found to be effective at reducing pain and leg oedema, although its efficacy and safety in the long-term has not been studied. Some plant extract like the α-benzopyronecoumarin are effective venoactive drugs, although its use has been limited due to its hepatotoxicity (Schmeck-Lindenau HJ *et al*, 2003). Other natural venoactive drugs, like *Ginkgo biloba* extract, ruscus extracts, etc., have been evaluated, even though their benefits are limited and the available evidence is considered insufficient to support their routine use (reviewed in Gohel MS *et al*, 2009).

Synthetic venoactive drugs like calcium dobesilate, that had shown promising results in preliminary studies (Gohel MS *et al*, 2010), showed no significant short-term effects in a multicenter randomized study that counted with the participation of our group (Martínez-Zapata MJ *et al*, 2008), therefore more studies are needed to evaluate its sustained effect and to support its use.

3.2.2. Non-Venoactive Agents

Non-venoactive drugs have been used mainly to treat patients with venous ulcers. Several adjuvant non-venoactive drugs with anti-inflammatory properties have been used to stimulate and accelerate ulcer healing (reviewed in Gohel MS *et al*, 2010).

3.2.2.1. Prostaglandin E₁

Prostaglandin E1 (PGE_1) has a number of effects on the microcirculation, including reduction of leukocyte activation, platelet aggregation inhibition, small vessel vasodilatation and reduction of levels of vessel wall cholesterol. Several studies in the 1980's demonstrated its beneficial effects in the treatment of CVD (Beitner H *et al*, 1980; Rudofsky G *et al*, 1989). A more recent study demonstrated the effectiveness of PGE_1 in reducing the healing time of venous ulcers; in addition, the drug has the advantage of being well tolerated by the patients and its side effects are acceptable (Milio G *et al*.2005)

3.2.2.2. Prostacyclin Analogues

Iloprost (Schering, Berlin), a synthetic prostacyclin analogue with the capacity to increase fibrinolytic activity, has been used with success in the treatment of peripheral vascular disease like arterial and diabetic ulcers (Müller B et al, 1988; Musial J et al, 1986). In addition to its better-known effects on platelet behaviour, it has profound effects on leucocyte activity by reducing adhesion to endothelium (Belch JJF et al, 1987). However, in a double blind, placebo controlled study, no improvement for venous leg ulcers was found with the topical use of iloprost (Werner-Schlenzka H et al, 1994)

3.2.2.3. Pentoxifylline

It is thought that pentoxifylline mechanism of action might include the improvement of red cell deformability and the subsequent oxygen delivery to ischemic tissue, as well as inhibition of leukocyte adhesion to endothelium and the release of superoxide free radicals produced in the so-called respiratory burst characteristic of neutrophil degranulation (Sullivan GW et al, 1988). Since 1989, pentoxifylline has been evaluated in several trials and promising results were initially obtained (Angelides NS et al, 1989). In fact, statistically significant effect on ulcer healing was obtained in a multi-centre placebo-controlled double-blind prospective study of 80 patients treated with 1200 mg/day of pentoxifylline for six months (Colgan MP et al, 1990). However, when used in combination with compression therapy, even though a trend towards more rapid healing in the pentoxifylline group was observed, this did not reach statistical significance (Dale JJ et al, 1999).

3.2.2.4.Acetylsalicylic Acid (ASA)

An in vitro study using segments of vein excised at surgery from patients treated with either low dose of aspirin, 25 mg per day, or placebo, suggested that this drug might have certain therapeutic benefits due to its anti-aggregating properties, by a mechanism involving prostacyclin production from the vascular endothelium (Costantini V et al, 1990). Few studies have been reported to test the effectiveness of aspirin and platelet antagonists in venous ulceration, most likely due the absence of commercial exploitation. The use of aspirin in a clinical study was reported in 1994 (Layton A et al, 1994), although the effect of aspirin on the rate of ulcer healing did not provide valid conclusions. A randomized controlled study using a potent blocker of the platelet function, TXA_2, showed no effect on leg ulcer healing (Lyon RT, 1998), arguing for a target of aspirin other than the anti-platelet effect. Other studies have suggested the existence of alterations in coagulation in patients with CVD, i.e., fibrinogen, factor VIII, von Willebrand antigen and activator inhibitor-1 (PAI-1), which can be modified by the use of aspirin (Ibbotson SH *et al*, 1995). Recent findings from our group have shown that treatment of patients with varicose syndrome with higher doses of ASA, 300 mg per day, accelerated healing and delayed recurrence of venous ulceration (Del Rio Sola ML *et al*, in press), suggesting that anti-inflammatory properties of aspirin not linked to inhibition of platelet activation could explain the observed effect. More studies are needed, but these observations suggest that ASA could be used as complementary treatment for CVD.

3.2.2.5.Synthetic Peptide

Thymosin β4 (Tβ4), a G-actin-sequestering molecule, has been found to have wound healing and anti-inflammatory properties, including the induction of cell migration, blood vessel formation, cell survival, the modulation of cytokines and specific proteases, and the upregulation of matrix molecules. A phase 2 study have shown promising results since a Tβ4 dose of 0.03% has the potential to accelerate wound healing and that complete wound healing can be achieved within 3 months in about 25% of the patients, being specially effective in small and moderate wounds (Guarnera G *et al*, 2010). As for the mechanism, it is thought to exert its therapeutic effect through promotion of keratinocyte and endothelial cell migration, increased collagen deposition, and stimulation of angiogenesis.

3.2.3. Other Potential Pharmacological Agents

In the last few years, experimental studies with human tissues and animal models have emphasized the role of several inflammatory mediators in the pathogenesis of CVD and suggested that some of them could be used as potential therapeutic targets in the future.

Growth factors antagonists. Growth factors successfully improve wound repair in animal studies when applied topically (Pierce GF *et al*, 1989); however, similar studies on humans with venous leg ulcers have not been successful. In addition, since the increase of VEGF level parallels with the severity of CVD (Howlader MH *et al*, 2004), it has been proposed that the use of inhibitors designed to block VEGF could be beneficial to treat CVD (Schmid-Schönbein G, 2007). More recently, a phase I study demonstrated the initial safety, feasibility, and biologic plausibility of using peri-ulcer injection of a replication-incompetent adenoviral construct expressing PDGF-β to treat venous leg ulcer disease (Margolis DJ *et al*, 2009).

MMPs modulators. MMPs play an important role on the remodeling of the extracellular matrix characteristic of the CVD, and the ratio MMPs/TIMPs could be a potential therapeutic target (Raffetto JD *et al*, 2008). In fact, MMP modulators have been used for several clinical applications (Raffetto JD *et al*, 2008). The use of synthetic pharmacological inhibitors of TIMPs such as BB-94 (Batimastat) and doxycycline, and Ro-28-2653, a more specific inhibitor of gelatinases and MMP-1, could be beneficial in reducing the MMP-mediated vascular dysfunction and the progressive vessel wall damage associated with vascular diseases (Raffetto JD *et al*, 2008).

Chemokine antagonists. Elevated expression of chemokines has been reported as a hallmark of varicose vein disease (Del Rio Sola ML *et al*, 2009). In the same study, it was observed that the treatment with aspirin during 2 weeks before surgery of CVD patients had a trend towards diminishing the elevated levels of chemokines in varicose veins, but the effect did not reach a statistical significance (Del Rio Sola ML *et al*, 2009). One explanation is that the dose, 300 mg of aspirin per day that was chosen for its benefit on ulcer healing (Del Rio Sola ML *et al*, in press), was lower than that used for inflammatory diseases and required for reduction of chemokine expression *in vitro*. Another explanation is that the duration of the treatment was insufficient to achieve a significant effect. Even though more studies are needed, our data suggest that pharmacological therapy aimed at reducing chemokine expression may have a role in the management of venous diseases in the future (Del Rio Sola ML *et al*, 2009; Del Rio Sola ML *et al*, in press).

HIF inhibitors. HIF-1α and HIF-2α have been associated to CVD, and based on recent evidence it is thought that drugs designed to block HIFs might have a beneficial effects on the treatment of CVD (Lim CS *et al*, 2011a).

CONCLUSION

Although the cause and sequences of events that occur during the development and progression of CVD have not completely been elucidated, both disturbed venous-flow patterns and chronic inflammation may underlie all the clinical manifestations of the disease. Therefore, treatment at the early stages of the disease designed to prevent inflammation could alleviate symptoms of chronic venous disease and reduce the risk of ulcers. Many of the currently available drugs can attenuate various components of the inflammatory cascade, particularly leukocyte-endothelium interactions. Improved understanding of the cellular and molecular mechanisms involved in the inflammation cascades underlying the CVD may allow the identification of potential therapeutic targets for pharmacological intervention. These potential anti-inflammatory drugs could be complementary to the current therapies that treat CVD. Animal models could be useful not only to study the early stages of the disease, but also to test the effects of new potential therapies, since they can reproduce some of the symptoms and features of varicosities in humans (Bergan JJ *et al*, 2008). More importantly, well-designed, large and high-quality clinical trials will be needed to evaluate the actual clinical benefits of potential anti-inflammatory drugs, either alone or in combination with current therapies for the treatment of CVD.

DECLARATION

The authors declare no conflict of interest.

REFERENCES

Ahti TM, Mäkivaara LA, Luukkaala T, Hakama M, Laurikka JO.Effect of family history on the incidence of varicose veins: a population-based follow-up study in Finland. *Angiology.* 2009;60:487-91.

Angelides NS, Weil von der Ahe, CA. Effect of oral pentoxifylline therapy on venous lower extremity ulcers due to deep venous incompetence. *Angiology* 1989;40:752-763.

Aravind B, Saunders B, Navin T, Sandison A, Monaco C, Paleolog EM, Davies AH. Inhibitory Effect of TIMP Influences the Morphology of Varicose Veins. *Eur. J. Vasc.Endovasc. Surg.* 2010; 40:754-65.

Badier-Commander C, Verbeuren T, Lebard C, Michel JB, Jacob MP. Increased TIMP/MMP ratio in varicose veins: a possible explanation for extracellular matrix accumulation. *J. Pathol.* 2000;192:105-112.

Balmer A, Limoni C. A double-blind placebo-controlled trial of VENORUTON on the symptoms and signs of chronic venous insufficiency. *Vasa* 1980;9:76-82.

Beidler SK, Douillet CD, Berndt DF, Keagy BA, Rich PB, Marston WA.Inflammatory cytokine levels in chronic venous insufficiency ulcer tissue before and after compression therapy. *J. Vasc. Surg.* 2009;49:1013-20.

Beitner H, Hammar H, Olsson AG and Thyresson N. Prostaglandin E1 treatment of leg ulcers caused by venous or arterial incompetence. *Acta Derm Venereol.* 1980;60:425-430.

Belch JJF, Saniabadi A, Dickson R, Sturrock RD and Forbes CD. Effect of Iloprost (ZK 36374) on white cell behaviour. In: Gryglewski RJ and Stock G, eds. Prostacyclin and its Stable Analogue Iloprost. Berlin: Springer-Verlag, 1987:97-102.

Bergan JJ, Schmid-Schonbein GW, Coleridge-Smith PD, Nicolaides AN, Boisseau MR, Eklof B. Chronic venous disease. *N. Engl. J. Med.* 2006;355:488-98.

Bergan J, Pascarella L, Schmid-Schönbein GW. Pathogenesis of primary chronic venous disease: insights from animal models of venous hypertension. *J. Vasc.Surg.* 2008;47:183-192.

Boisseau M. Effect of shear stress in vascular endothelial changes. *Phlebolymphology* 2003; 40:143-55.

Boisseau MR. Leukocyte involvement in the signs and symptoms of chronic venous disease.Perspectives for therapy. *Clin. Hemorheol. Microcirc.* 2007;37:277-290.

Cario-Toumaniantz C, Boularan C, Schurgers LJ, Heymann MF, Le Cunff M, Léger J, Loirand G, Pacaud P. Identification of differentially expressed genes in human varicose veins: involvement of matrix gla protein in extracellular matrix remodeling. *J. Vasc. Res.* 2007;44:444-59.

Bujan J, Jurado F, Gimeno MJ. Changes in metalloproteases expression (MMP-1, MMP-2) in the proximal region of the varicose saphenous vein in young subjects. *Phebology.* 2000;15: 64-70.

Charles CA, Romanelli P, Martinez ZB, Ma F, Roberts B, KirsnerRS.Tumor necrosis factor-alpha in nonhealing venous leg ulcers. *J. Am. Acad. Dermatol.* 2009;60:951-5.

Coleridge-Smith PD, Thomas P, Scurr JH, Dormandy JA. Causes of venous ulceration: a new hypothesis. *Br. Med. J.* 1988;296:1726-7.

Coleridge-Smith PD. Deleterious effects of white cells in the course of skin damage in CVD. *Angiology.*1997;48:77-85.

Coleridge-Smith P, Bergan JJ. Inflammation in venous disease. In: Schmid-Schonbein G, Granger DN, editors. Molecular basis for microcirculatory disorders. Paris: Springer; 2003. p. 489-513.

Colgan M-P, Dormandy JA, Jones PW, Schraibman IG, Shanik DG and Young RAL. Oxpentifylline treatment of venous ulcers of the leg. *Br. Med. J.* 1990; 300:972-975.

Costantini V, Talpacci A, Cipolloni S, Boschetti E, Bisacci R, Tristaino B, Nenci GG. Effect of aspirin and dipyridamole treatment on prostacyclin production by human veins. *Thromb. Res.* 1990;58:109-17.

Dale JJ, Ruckley CV, Harper DR, Gibson B, Nelson EA, Prescott RJ. A randomised double-blind placebo controlled trial of pentoxifylline in the treatment of venous leg ulcers. *BMJ.* 1999;319:875-8.

Deatrick K, Wakefield T, Henke P. Chronic venous insufficiency: current management of varicose vein disease. *Am. Surg.* 2010;76:125-32.

De Jongste AB, Jonker JJC, Huisman MV, Ten Cate JW, Azar AJ. A double blind three center clinical trial on the short-term efficacy of O-(b-hydroxyethyl)-rutosides in patients with post-thrombotic syndrome. *Thromb. Haemost.* 1989;62:826-829.

Del Rio Sola ML, Aceves M, Dueñas AI, González-Fajardo JA, Vaquero C, Sánchez Crespo M, García-Rodríguez C. Varicose veins show enhanced chemokine expression. *Eur.Vasc.Endovasc. Surg.* 2009;38:635-641.

Del Río-Solá L, González-Fajardo JA, Vaquero, Puerta C. Influence of acetylsalicylic acid therapy in ulcer associated with chronic venous insufficiency. *Ann Vasc.Surg.* In press.

Eberhardt RT, Rafetto JD. Chronic venous insufficiency. *Circulation.* 2005;111:2398-409.

Eklof B, Perrin M, Delis KT, Rutherford RB, Gloviczki P. Updated terminology of chronic venous disorders: The VEIN-TERM transatlantic interdisciplinary consensus document. *J. Vasc. Surg.* 2009;49:498-501

Evans CJ, Fowkes FG, Ruckley CV, Lee AJ. Prevalence of varicose veins and chronic venous insufficiency in men and women in the general population: Edinburgh Vein Study. *J. Epidemiol. Community Health.* 1999;53:149-53.

Fiebig A, Krusche P, Wolf A, Krawczak M, Timm B, Nikolaus S, Frings, Schreiber S. Heritability of chronic venous disease. *Hum. Genet.* 2010;127:669-74.

Fukuda S, Yasu T, Predescu DN, Schmid-Schonbein GW. Mechanisms for regulation of fluid shear stress response in circulating leucocytes. *Circ. Res.* 2000;86:E13-8.

Ghaderian SM, Lindsey NJ, Graham AM, Homer-Vanniassinkam S and AkbarzadehNajar R. Pathogenic mechanisms in varicose vein disease: the role of hypoxia and inflammation. *Pathology.* 2010;42:446–453.

Gloviczki P, Gloviczki ML.Evidence on efficacy of treatments of venous ulcers and on prevention of ulcer recurrence. *Perspect Vasc. Surg.Endovasc.Ther.*2009;21:259-68

Gohel MS, Windhaber RAJ, Tarlton JFT, Whyman MR, Poskitt KR. The relationship between cytokine concentrations and wound healing in chronic venous ulceration. *J. Vasc. Surg.* 2008;48:1272-1277.

Gohel MS, Davies AH. Pharmacological agents in the treatment of venous disease: an update of the available evidence. *Curr. Vasc. Pharmacol.* 2009;7:301-308.

Gohel MS, Davies AH. Pharmacological treatment of C4, C5 and C6 venous disease. *Phlebology.* 2010;25:S35-41.

Guarnera G, DeRosa A, Camerini R; 8 European sites.The effect of thymosin treatment of venous ulcers. *Ann. N. Y. Acad. Sci.* 2010;1194:207-12.

Guilhou JJ, Dereure O, Marzin L, Ouvry P, Zuccarelli F, Debure C, *et al.* Efficacy of Daflon 500 mg in venous leg ulcer healing: a double-blind, randomised, controlled versus placebo trial in 107 patients. *Angiology.* 1997;48:77-85.

Haynes DF, Kerstein MD, Roberts MP, Bell WH 3rd, Rush DS, Kadowitz PJ, McNamara DB.Increased prostacyclin and thromboxane A2 formation in human varicose veins. *J. Surg. Res.* 1990;49:228-32.

Ibbotson SH, Layton AM, Davies JA, Goodfield MJ. The effect of aspirin on haemostatic activity in the treatment of chronic venous leg ulceration. *Br. J. Dermatol.*1995; 132:422-6.

Jacob MP, Badier-Commander C, Fontaine V, Benazzoug Y, Feldman L, Michel JB. Extracellular matrix remodeling in the vascular wall. *Pathol. Biol.* 2001;49:326-32.

Junger M, Steins A, Hahn M, Hafner HM. Microcirculatory dysfunction in chronic venous insufficiency (CVD). *Microcirculation.* 2000;7:S3-S12.

Kakkos SK, Zolota VG, Peristeropoulou P, Apostolopoulou A, Geroukalos G, Tsolakis IA. Increased mast cell infiltration in familial varicose veins: pathogenetic implications? *Int.Angiol.* 2003;22:43-9.

Karatepe O, UnalO,Ugurlucan M, Kemik A, Karahan S, Aksoy M and Kurtoglu M. The impact of valvular oxidative stress on the development of venous stasis ulcer valvular oxidative stress and venous ulcers. *Angiology.* 2010;61:283-288.

Kendler M, Makrantonaki E, Tzellos T, Kratzsch J, Anderegg U, Wetzig T, Zouboulis C, Simon JC. Elevated sex steroid hormones in great saphenous veins in men. *J. Vasc. Surg.* 2010;51:639-46.

Kowalewski R, Malkowski A, Sobolewski K, Gacko M. Evaluation of transforming growth factor-beta signaling pathway in the wall of normal and varicose veins. *Pathobiology.* 2010;77:1-6.

Layton A, Ibbotson S, Davies JA, Goodfield M. Randomised trial of oral aspirin for chronic venous leg ulcers. *Lancet.* 1994; 344:164-5.

Lim CS, Gohel MS, Shepherd AC, Paleolog E, Davies AH. Venous hypoxia: A poorly studied ethiological factor of varicose veins. *J. Vasc. Res.* 2011;48:185-194 (a).

Lim CS, Qiao X, Reslan O, Xia Y, Raffetto JD, Paleolog E, Davies AH, Khalil RA. Prolonged mechanical stretch is associated with upregulation of hypoxia-inducible factors and reduced contraction in rat inferior vena cava. *J.Vasc. Surg.* 2011;53:764-73 (b)

Lyon RT, Veith FJ, Bolton L, Machado F. Clinical benchmark for healing of chronic venous ulcers. Venous Ulcer Study Collaborators. *Am. J. Surg.* 1998 Aug;176:172-5.

Makino A, Prossnitz ER, Bünemann M, Wang JM, Yao W, Schmid-Schönbein GW. G protein-coupled receptors serve as mechanosensors for fluid shear stress in neutrophils. *Am. J. Physiol. Cell Physiol.* 2006;290:C1633-9.

Margolis DJ, Morris LM, Papadopoulos M, Weinberg L, Filip JC, Lang SA, Vaikunth SS, Crombleholme TM. Phase I study of H5.020CMV.PDGF-beta to treat venous leg ulcer disease. *Mol. Ther.* 2009;17:1822-9.

Martínez-Zapata MJ, Moreno RM, Gich I, Urrútia G, Bonfill X; Chronic Venous Insufficiency Study Group. A randomized, double-blindmulticentre clinical trial comparing the efficacy of calcium dobesilate with placebo in the treatment of chronic venous disease. *Eur. J. Vasc. Endovasc. Surg.* 2008;35:358-65.

Michiels C, Arnould T, Remacle J. Endothelial cell responses to hypoxia: initiation of a cascade of cellular interactions. *Biochem. Biophys. Acta.* 2000; 1497:1-10.

Milio G, Minà C, Cospite V, Almasio PL, Novo S. Efficacy of the treatment with prostaglandin E-1 in venous ulcers of the lower limbs. *J. Vasc. Surg.* 2005;42:304-8.

Moazzam F, Delano FA, Zweifach BW, Schmid-Schönbein GW.The leucocyte response to fluid stress. *Proc. Natl. Acad. Sci.* USA. 1997;94:13152-7.

Müller B, Krais T, Sturzebacher S, Witt W, Schillinger E and Baldus B. Potential therapeutic mechanisms of stable prostacyclin (PGI2) mimetics in severe peripheral vascular disease. *Biomed. Biochim. Acta.* 1988;47:S40-44.

Murphy MA, Joyce WP, Condron C, Bouchier-Hayes D. A reduction in serum *Eur. J.Vasc. Endovasc. Surg.* 2002;23:349-52.

Musial J, Wilczynska M, Sladek K, Ciernewski CS, Nizankowski R and Szczeklik A. Fibrinolytic activity of prostacyclin and Iloprost in patients with peripheral arterial disease. *Prostaglandins*.1986;31:61-70

Nicolaides AN. Chronic venous disease and the leukocyte endothelium interaction: from symptoms to ulceration. *Angiology.* 2005;56:S11-S19.

Nocker W, Diebschlag W and Lehmacher W. Clinical trials of the dose-related effects of O-(ß-hydroxyethyl)-rutosides in patients with chronic venous insufficiency. *Phlebology. 1990; 5:23-26.*

O'Donnell TF, Lau J. A systematic review of randomized controlled trials of wound dressings for chronic venous ulcer. *J.Vasc. Surg.* 2006;44:1118-25.

Ono T, Bergan JJ, Schmid-Schönbein GN, Takase S. Monocyte infiltration into venous valves. *J.Vasc. Surg.* 1998;27:158-166.

Pappas PJ, DeFouw DO, Venezio LM, et al. Morphometric assessment of the dermal microcirculation in patients with chronic venous insufficiency. *J. Vasc. Surg.* 1997; 26:784-95.

Pappas PJ, You R, Rameshwar P, Gorti R, DeFouw DO, Phillips CK, Padberg FT Jr, Silva MB Jr, Simonian GT, Hobson RW 2nd, Durán WN. Dermal tissue fibrosis in patients with chronic venous insufficiency is associated with increased transforming growth factor-beta1 gene expression and protein production. *J. Vasc. Surg.* 1999;30:1129-45.

Pappas PJ, Brajesh K L, Padberg TF. Pathophysiology of chronic venous disease. In: The Vein Book. Ed. John Bergan, Canada, Elsevier 2007, p.89-101.

Pascarella L, Lulic D, Penn AH, Alsaigh T, Lee J, Shin H, Kapur V, Bergan JJ, Schmid-Schönbein GW. Mechanisms in experimental venous valve failure and their modification by Daflon 500 mg. *Eur. J. Vasc. Endovasc. Surg.* 2008;35:102-10.

Pastar I, Stojadinovic O, Krzyzanowska A, Barrientos S, Stuelten C, Zimmerman K, Blumenberg M, Brem H, Tomic-Canic M. Attenuation of the transforming growth factor beta-signaling pathway in chronic venous ulcers. *Mol. Med.* 2010;16:92-101.

Perrot-Applanat M, Cohen-Solal K, Milgrom E, Finet M. Progesterone receptor expression in human saphenous veins. *Circulation.* 1995;92:2975-83.

Pierce GF, Mustoe TA, Lingelbach J, Masakowski VR, Griffin GL, Senior RM, Deuel TF. Platelet-derived growth factor and transforming growth factor-beta enhance tissue repair activities by unique mechanisms. *J. Cell Biol.* 1989;109:429-40.

Pulvertaft TB. General practice treatment of symptoms of venous insufficiency with oxerutins.Results of a 660 patient multicentre study in the UK. *Vasa*.1983;12:373-376.

Raffetto JD, Ross RL, Khalil RA. Matrix metalloproteinase 2-induced venous dilation via hyperpolarization and activation of K+ channel: Relevance to varicose vein formation. *J. Vas. Surg.* 2007;45:373-380.

Raffetto JD. Chronic venous insufficiency: molecular abnormalities and ulcer formation. In: The Vein Book. Ed. John Bergan, Canada, Elsevier 2007, 79-87.

Raffetto JD, Khalil RA.Matrix metalloproteinases and their inhibitors in vascular remodeling and vascular disease. *Biochem.Pharmacol.* 2008;75:346-59.

Raffetto JD, Qiao X, Beauregard KG, Khalil RA. Estrogen receptor-mediated enhancement of venous relaxation in female rat: implications in sex-related differences in varicose veins. *J. Vasc. Surg.* 2010;51:972-81.

Rudofsky G. Intravenous prostaglandin E1 in the treatment of venous ulcers - a double-blind, placebo-controlled trial. *Vasa*. 1989; 28:S39-43.

Saharay M, Shields DA, Porter JB, Scurr JH, Coleridge Smith PD. Leukocyte activity in the microcirculation of the leg in patients with chronic venous disease. *J. Vasc. Surg.*1997;26:265-73.

Saharay M, Shields DA, Georgiannos SN, Porter JB, Scurr JH, Coleridge Smith PD. Endothelial activation in patients with chronic venous disease *Eur. J. Vasc. Endovasc. Surg.* 1998;15:342-9

Sansilvestri-Morel P, Rupin A, Badier-Commander C, Kern P, Fabiani JN, Verbeuren TJ, Vanhoutte PM. Imbalance in the synthesis of collagen type I and collagen type III in smooth muscle cells derived from human varicose veins. *J.Vasc. Res.* 2001;38:560-8.

Sansilvestri-Morel P, Rupin A, Badier-Commander C, Fabiani JN, Verbeuren TJ. Chronic venous insufficiency: dysregulation of collagen synthesis. *Angiology.* 2003; 54:S13-8.

Satokawa H, Hoshino S, Igari T, Iwaya F, Midorikawa H. The appearance of cytokines and adhesion molecules in saphenous vein valves in chronic venous insuciency. *Phlebology.* 2002;16: 106-10.

Schmid-Schonbein G, Takase S, Bergan JJ. New advances in the understanding of the pathophysiology of chronic venous insufficiency. *Angiology.* 2001;52:S27-8.

Schmid-Schönbein G. Molecular basis of venous insufficiency. In: The Vein Book. Ed. John Bergan, Canada, Elsevier 2007, p. 67-78.

Schmid-Schönbein, G. Triggering mechanisms of venous valve incompetence. *Medicographia.* 2008;30; 121-126

Schmeck-Lindenau HJ, Naser-Hijazi B, Becker EW, Henneicke-von Zepelin HH, Schnitker J. Safety aspects of a coumarin-troxerutin combination regarding liver function in a double-blind placebo-controlled study. *Int. J. Clin. Pharmacol. Ther.* 2003;41:193-9.

Shields DA, Andaz SK, Sarin S, Scurr JH, Coleridge Smith PD. Plasma elastase in venous disease. *Br. J. Surg.* 1994;81:1496-9.

Shoab SS, Scurr JH, Coleridge-Smith PD. Increased plasma vascular endothelial growth factor among patients with chronic venous disease. *J. Vasc. Surg.* 1998;28:535-40.

Somers P, Knaapen M. The Histopathology of varicose vein disease. *Angiology.* 2006;57:546-55.

Sprague A, Khalil R. Inflammatory cytokines in vascular dysfunction and vascular disease. *Biochem. Pharmacol.* 2009;78:539-552.

Sullivan GW, Carper HT, Novick WJ andMandell GL. Inhibition of the inflammatory action of interleukin-1 and tumour necrosis factor (alpha) on neutrophil function by pentoxifylline. *Infect.Immunol.* 1988;56:1722-1729.

Takase S, Schmid-Schönbein G, Bergan JJ. Leukocyte activation in patients with venous insufficiency. *J. Vasc. Surg.*1999;30:148-156.

Takase S, Bergan JJ, Schmid-Schönbein GW. Expression of adhesion molecules and cytokines on saphenous veins in chronic venous insufficiency. *Ann .Vasc. Surg.* 2000;14:427-435.

Tanaka H, Zaima N, Yamamoto N, Sagara D, Suzuki M, Nishiyama M, Mano Y, Sano M, Hayasaka T, Goto-Inoue N, Sasaki T, Konno H, Unno N, Setou M. *Eur. J. Vasc. Endovasc. Surg.* 2010;40:657-63.

Thomas PR, Nash GB, Dormandy JA. White cell accumulation in dependent legs of patients with venous hypertension: a possible mechanism for trophic changes in the skin. *Br. Med. J.* 1988;296:1693-5.

Werner-Schlenzka H, Kuhlmann RK. Treatment of venous leg ulcers with topical Iloprost: a placebo controlled study. *Vasa.* 1994;23:145-50.

Wilms H, Delano FA and Schmid-Schönbein GW. Mechanisms of parenchymal cell death in-vivo after microvascularhemorrhage. *Microcirculation.* 2000;7,1–11.

Woodside KJ, Hu M, Burke A, *et al.* Morphologic characteristics of varicose veins: possible role of metalloproteinases. *J. Vasc. Surg.* 2003;38:162-169.

Yamakawa Y, Takano M, Patel M, Tien N, Takada T, Bulkley GB. Interaction of platelet activating factor, reactive oxygen species generated by xanthine oxidase, and leukocytes in the generation of hepatic injury after shock/resuscitation. *Ann. Surg.* 2000;231:387-98.

Yong K, Khwaja A. Leukocyte cellular adhesion molecules. *Blood Rev.* 1990;4:211-25.

Zimmerman GA, McIntyre TM, Prescott SM. Adhesion and signaling in vascular cell-cell interactions. *J. Clin. Invest.* 1996;98:1699-702.

In: Varicose Veins   ISBN 978-1-61209-841-8
Editor: Andrea L. Nelson   © 2011 Nova Science Publishers, Inc.

Chapter 3

ASCENDING EVOLUTION OF VARICOSE VEINS: LITERATURE REVIEW AND RATIONALE FOR TREATMENT

Paola De Rango[1,1], Bernardini Eugenio[2],
Paolo Bonanno[1] and Deborah Brambilla[1]
[1]Vascular Endovascular Surgery, Hospital S.M. Misericordia,
Perugia, Italy
[2]Centro Ricerche Cliniche Università di Camerino
Macerata, Italy

ABSTRACT

Partially due to the lack and difficulty in conducting longitudinal studies on the natural history of primary varicose veins, the pathophysiologic mechanisms that lead to the development and progression of vein reflux in lower limbs is unknown. Increasing evidence suggests that the development of primary venous insufficiency can follow an ascending pattern where the terminal valve is the last to be involved. This is conflicting with the traditional "retrograde" theory stating that the incompetence of valves above the saphenofemoral junction is the primary source of varicose disease that proceeds in a

[1] Corresponding Author: Paola De Rango, MD, Vascular and Endovascular Unit, Hospital S.M. Misericordia, University of Perugia, 06129, Perugia, Italy. Phone: +39 075-5786440. Fax: +39 075-5786435. Email: plderango@gmail.com, pderango@unipg.it.

retrograde manner with progressive dilatation and valvular incompetence along the saphenous vein (SV) and its tributaries.

The ascending evolution is supported by hemodynamic principles, literature data and direct observations.

1. According to scientific laws, the development of venous insufficiency in lower limb is likely determined by the hydrostatic column of venous pressure and thereby follows the gravity gradient along the column. The lower the level (higher the gravity force), the higher the hydrostatic pressure causing venous incompetence and the reflux to begin. Once started a lower point, varicose vein disease can subsequently evolve uprising in accordance with the pressure gradient.
2. There is evidence to support that terminal valve involvement in varicose disease of SV can occur in less half population with SV insufficiency . In 45-55% of cases refluxes along SV are found below competent terminal valves that are therefore last components of SV to be involved from venous insufficiency.
3. Studies using selective and minimally invasive approach to treat varicose veins have also shown that after treatment localized in a target vein, the shrinkage and recovery of the of dilated varicose vein above can occur. This could not be explained with a retrograde development of varicose disease where the disease at above levels was antecedent and prelude to the involvement of lower venous segments.

The natural history of varicose veins is that of a progressive disease which chronic evolution. Although the exact development is uncertain, it is likely that the disease begins at the lower levels of the limbs and develops in an antegrade manner as venous stasis is higher where force of gravity is higher. This data do not support an aggressive and widespread treatment of the saphenous terminal valve as first strategy in the presence of varicose veins of lower limbs.

INTRODUCTION

Primary Varicose veins are a common medical condition that may affect 5%-30% of adult population of western industrialized countries with significant impact on individual's health and health care system.[1-2] Female predominate by a ratio between 1.3:1 and 4.0:1. The annual incidence of the pathology is about 1.0% in men and 1.3% in women; however, estimates of prevalence vary among epidemiology studies because of differences in the classification or definition used, methods of evaluation, populations and geographic region studied. Studies indicate a prevalence of 10-15% of men and 20-25% of women but, when milder forms of varicosities are also included, the estimated prevalence raises to approximately 45% in men and 50% in women.[2-4] The prevalence further increases with age rising from approximately 25% at age of 30 years to more than 60% at age of 70 years. The etiology of primary varicose vein is known as an interaction of predisposing factors (the major being the weakness of the smooth muscle of the vein wall that may be an inherited condition or, more often, a primary factor, especially in women) and a number of manifestation factors, including age, height, pregnancy, prolonged standing, dietary habits, body posture and overweight.

Despite the large diffusion of the disease and the significant burden on health care resources, due to both cosmetic appearance and associated symptoms (especially in advanced stages), the physiology and pathogenesis leading to primary varicose veins are still object of debate. There is no doubt that primary varicose vein represents a chronic evolving disorder with inevitable deterioration over time. Nevertheless, the exact mechanisms behind the development and progression of the disease have not been completely elucidated. This mainly because of the difficulty in conducting large longitudinal epidemiology studies to understand the natural history of a common condition that is however demanding to follow in standardized settings due to notably difference in distribution, severity, populations, treatments and compliance of patients. Due to the lack of such longitudinal evidence on the natural history, the hypotheses on pathophysiology mechanisms responsible for progression of reflux in primary superficial venous insufficiency remain often based on personal view points and, therefore, largely uncertain. Critical analysis of evidence resulting from each of the formulated assumptions is relevant since different theoretical models also provide a valuable and necessary basis for the development of new and improvement of existing therapy.

PATHOPHYSIOLOGY OF VARICOSE VEINS AND "RETROGRADE THEORY"

Venous pathology develops when venous pressure is increased and return of blood is impaired through several mechanisms including valve incompetence and muscle pump dysfunction. These mechanisms induce venous hypertension particularly when standing or ambulating. With dysfunction or incompetence of the valves in the superficial venous system, the blood is pumped out of the extremities but refill occurs (because of retrograde venous flow) along with development of increased hydrostatic pressure. In primary superficial venous varicosities, valve failure generally occurs as a result of preexisting weakness in the vessel wall or valve leaflets; nevertheless valve incompetence may also be secondary to direct injury, superficial phlebitis or excessive venous distention from high pressure. The traditional long-held "Trendelemburg" theory of development and propagation of venous insufficiency was based on the belief that the common starting point for any varicosity is a pressure and volume overload on one segment of a superficial vein located distal to an incompetent valve at a point where the superficial venous system drains into the deep system. According to this theory, venous dilatation and varicose veins are though to form and propagate from the terminal valve to the extremities following a progressive descending valvular incompetence. Thus, the junctional valve of a saphenous vein is incompetent first, while only after this occurrence and because the venous pressure in the lower limbs is increased in the upright posture due to hydrostatic reasons, the reflux develops along the vein in a retrograde manner: the thigh portions of the saphenous vein are affected first and, over time, there is a tendency for the changes to progress toward the periphery. Once the varicosities have produced certain degree of hemodynamic changes, the progression becomes self-sustaining. The traditional theory was therefore based on the belief that valve incompetence was the primary cause of venous varicosities with a "retrograde" propagation ("Retrograde theory") from above-to below levels along the leg. Failure of the valve located at the junction, most notably at saphenous-femoral and saphenous-popliteal junctions, allows high pressure to enter in the superficial veins and the progression to occur. This long-held Trendelemburg theory remains today still widely taught and accepted.[5-6]

Nevertheless, more recent data suggest that incompetent valves result from and are consequent to changes in the vein wall leading to dilatation of the vessels. As a consequence, development of venous insufficiency might not follow a retrograde route but multifocal and ascending patterns of venous insufficiency propagation have become indeed more likely suggested. This has led to the more recent "Ascending theory".

ASCENDING THEORY

1. Ascending Theory: Rationale and Theoretical Assumptions

From the "Ascending theory" view point, the terminal valve incompetence is not the starting point of primary varicose vein but the last to be reached. The theory was based on multiple morphology, biochemical, hemodynamic, and physic assumptions.

In the last years it has been consistently suggested that venous wall dilatation occurring in sites of venous reflux is due to morphology changes in collagen and elastin content and endothelial stem cell and does not have correlations with the site and function of valves. According to these findings, "wall weakening" is the initiating factor of primary reflux that, therefore, might not develop in a retrograde manner beginning from the terminal valve but, more likely, following a reverse, upward directed, or multifocal pattern. The theory on the "weakening" of the venous wall as the initiating factor of reflux has gained increasing support in many functional,morphological and biochemical studies.[7-9]

It is also known that even if varicose disease is associated with weakness of the vein wall, clinical manifestations occur only under certain orthostatic hemodynamic conditions. A primary wall abnormality (weakening) either along saphenous trunk or venous branches may be a predisposing factor necessary but not sufficient by itself to promote vein dilatation and reflux development in the absence of increased local pressure. Vein dilation under localized hyper-pressurization in turn produces veins valve incompetence, and the formation of a reflux that proceeds upwards according to the longitudinal distribution of local hydrostatic pressure weight. Hydrostatic columns of different heights create the necessary gradient for the development of reflux. Indeed, the hydrostatic column of venous pressure likely determines the natural history of primary venous insufficiency. Accordingly, the development of venous insufficiency in lower limbs should follow the gravity gradient: the lower the level, the higher the gravity force, the earlier the veins dilate (Laplace law), the valves separate and the reflux develops.

The Ascending theory is thereby based not only on theoretical and hemodynamic assumptions but also on physical laws.[10] The physiology of venous reflux explained as a retrograde phenomenon, as stated in the traditional theory, is poorly understandable since this does not agree with by basic physic principles and gravity force.

In assessing venous pressure in lower limbs, it should be recognized that the length and height of venous reflux is directly proportional to hydrostatic pressure (height of a column of water between the heart and ankle). The hydrostatic pressure gradient is directed downwards according to the gravity gradient (higher gravity at lower levels). Indeed, by static fluid laws, under the action of gravity a liquid exerts a resultant vertical force which equals the liquid weight; the pressure exerted by a static fluid depending on the depth of the fluid and the acceleration of gravity (Fluid Pressure Calculation [Fluid column height] in the relationship: $\Delta P = \rho g h$, where P=pressure, $\rho = m/V =$ fluid density, g = acceleration of gravity, h = depth of fluid]. Accordingly, venous stasis is higher at lower levels where force of gravity is higher.

Hemodynamic and physical principles therefore support that the natural history of venous insufficiency follows more likely an "ascending evolution" summarized as follows:

- Venous stasis is higher in the distal levels of the limbs where force of gravity is higher. Therefore, the reflux begins at the distal levels and vein dilatation with valve incompetence and reflux most likely begins at lower levels.
- The length and height of reflux is directly proportional to hydrostatic pressure (height of a column of water between the heart and ankle) and, accordingly, the pressure gradient is directed downwards (the highest pressure and the highest gradient at the bottom, the lowest pressure difference at the top of the column). Therefore, the reflux (once started) can subsequently develop in an antegrade fashion following the hydrostatic pressure gradient. That is, in the development of venous insufficiency, the lower the level, the higher the gravity force, the earlier the reflux develops and the veins dilate. The latest segment of the vein to be involved should be the terminal valve (i.e. SFJ, saphenous-popliteal junction) at the groin, due to the higher position along the hydrostatic column.

At the opposite, it is difficult to understand why should reflux develop in a retrograde manner, starting from the terminal valve or the thigh where the gravity and the pressure weight are lower and junction valves are intact (as demonstrated in more than half patients with primary venous insufficiency).[11-15] Favored by hydrostatic factors, primary venous insufficiency is most likely an ascending evolving disease.

The reversed view of the pathophysiology in development of primary venous reflux suggested by the "Ascending Theory" might be important also because of potential relevant implications for treatment, since clinical severity of varicosity generally is higher and more advanced at the starting points. To be effective, the most aggressive treatment should be driven at the lower starting levels, while the terminal valve most often does not require treatment. Furthermore, due to the segmental progression of venous disease, localized venous treatment at a lower level in an early stage of the disease could be applied to prevent the further progression of the disease to finally involve the terminal valve that can be indeed spared after treatment performed exclusively at a lower level.

Although the hypothesis of a non-retrograde evolution of primary venous insufficiency was recognized in the nineties, it was in the last more recent years, that there has been a growing renewed interest toward an "ascending" development of varicose veins. This interest was promoted by improvements in hemodynamic and ultrasound knowledge and by development of new opportunities to perform more conservative and selective treatments of varicose veins localized at the most severe and starting points of the disease.

2. Ascending Theory: Clinical Evidence

A number of studies have been published, to support this concept and data have been here reviewed. Unfortunately, there have been no studies large enough to provide strong evidence against the traditional retrograde evolution in the natural history of venous disease. In addition, published studies at this regard are not uniform, and heterogeneous populations have been analyzed. Difficulties in recruitment, assessment and following patients with symptoms or signs of venous insufficiency (most of them receiving one or more types of treatment misleading the natural evolution of the disease) obstacle the conduction of large population studies on this issue.

The rationale of the Ascending Theory is supported by a number of literature findings that can be included in 3 main fields of research in varicose veins:

a. Studies analyzing patterns/ distribution and progression of varicose veins. (Table I)
b. Studies investigating the prevalence of sapheno-femoral reflux at the junctions. (Table II)

    c.   Studies analyzing results and application of varicose veins treatments
          sparing the junctions / terminal valve. (Table III)

A. Clinical Data on Patterns of Venous Varicosities

Detailed analyses of patterns of varicosities distribution in lower limbs
suggested how the evolution of the disease might not follow a retrograde
propagation as early believed. Although there is a great variety in the patterns
of reflux and several papers have demonstrated variability in reflux patterns in
patients with vein insufficiency, it is known in clinical practice that the
appearance of varicosities in the medial and posteromedial aspect of the calf is
the most common reason for patients, especially women, to seek medical
attention. While not all the lower limbs varicosities involve the thigh and is
very uncommon to find isolated high thigh varicosities without lower calf
involvement. This assumption has been supported by a number of studies
analyzing the distribution and progression of varicose veins in different
population settings as summarized in Table I. Examples of varicose patterns
are shown in Figures 1-5.

PATTERNS OF REFLUX DEVELOPMENT

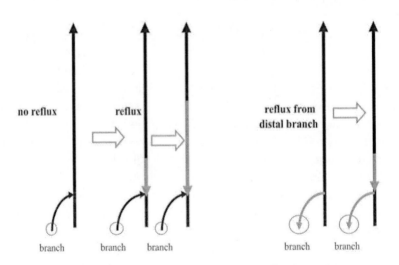

Figure 1. Different patterns of reflux development. On the left: reflux developed along
the saphenous trunk in ascending pattern. On the right: reflux developed from distal
tributary branch to saphenous trunk in ascending patterns.

Table I. Clinical data on patterns of venous varicosities

Authors	Year	Journal and title	Settings	Main findings	population
Reflux distribution and progression in non-treated limbs					
Labropoulos et al, [14]	1997	*Journal of Vascular Surgery* Where does venous reflux start?	Observational study on patterns of reflux in asymptomatic and patients with varicose veins	Significantly higher prevalence of reflux in calf saphenous veins (68%)than in the thigh (55%). Junction involved by reflux only in 32%	200
Labropoulos et al, [15]	2005	*Journal of Vascular Surgery* Study of the venous reflux progression.	Longitudinal observation of reflux in patients with varicose veins but without treatment	Reflux extension: antegrade and retrograde fashion; in continuity (14.7%) and separately (12.1%) from the preexisting disease (multi-focal)	116
Bernardini et al, [10]	2010	*Annals of Vascular Surgery* Development of primary superficial venous insufficiency: the ascending theory. Observational and hemodynamic data from a 9-year experience	Observation of venous patterns in primary superficial venous insufficiency left untreated	Progression in 94%. In 58% extension to one and in 42% progression to more than one above venous segments. No downward extension.	104
Reflux and Perforator veins					
Delis et al,[18]	2001	*Journal of Vascular Surgery* In situ hemodynamics of perforating veins in chronic venous insufficiency	Perforator veins reflux patterns	Incompetent thigh and lower-third calf perforators had significantly larger diameters than in the upper and middle calf (p<0.05)	265
Labropoulos et al , [19]	2006	*Journal of Vascular Surgery* Development of reflux in the perforator veins in limbs with primary venous disease	Perforator veins reflux patterns	Reflux in perforators veins developed in ascending fashion (47.4%) through superficial veins, at reentry points and at new sites	158
Reflux and tributaries veins					
Labropoulos et al, [22]	1999	*European Journal of Vascular Endovascular Surgery* Primary superficial vein reflux with competent saphenous trunk	Reflux patterns in patients with chronic venous disease without incompetence of saphenous trunk	Posterior arch tributaries veins of the calf most common involved: 46% Reflux only in tributaries below the knee: 28%	84

Table I. (Continued)

Authors	Year	Journal and title	Settings	Main findings	population
Engelhorn et al, [23]	2005	*Journal of Vascular Surgery* Patterns of saphenous reflux in women with primary varicose veins	Varicosities patterns in women with mild varicose disease	The large preponderance of varicose disease was distal and segmental. Along great saphenous vein (GSV) refluxing segments were noted most commonly in the leg (distal type) or in the leg and thigh (58%) while involvement of thigh was present in 37% and of junction only in 12% of cases	590

REFLUX DEVELOPMENT

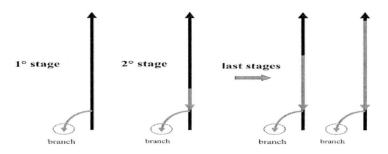

REFLUX DEVELOPMENT

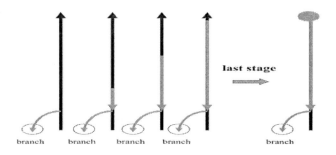

Figure 2. a and b. Longitudinal evolution of reflux in sequential patterns. Sequential patterns of reflux starting from a distal branch and developing along the saphenous trunk with ascending involvement. In Figure b, final involvement of the junction.

NON-SAPHENOUS VARICOSITY

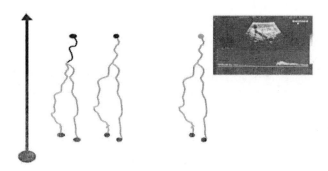

Figure 3. Non-saphenous varicosities with duplex pattern in the panel on the right.

REFLUX DEVELOPMENT

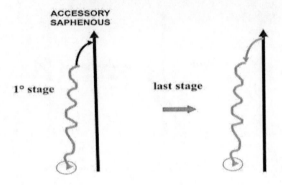

Figure 4. Reflux development along accessory saphenous vein.

INCOMPETENCE IN TRIBUTARY VEINS

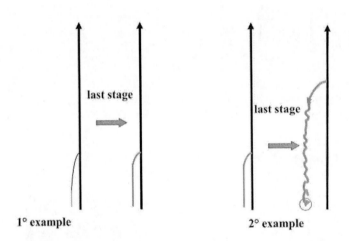

Figure 5. Examples of reflux ascending along tributary veins without saphenous trunk involvement. In both examples, from the First stage on the left toward the Last stage on the right

Reflux Distribution and Progression in Non-Treated Limbs

In 1997 Labropoulos et al.[14] published an observational study to identify the origin of lower limb primary venous reflux and to compare patterns of reflux in asymptomatic young individuals and matched subjects with clinical varicose veins. Overall 200 limbs were analyzed in three groups of patients: 40 in subjects with no symptoms, 40 in subjects with prominent but nonvaricose veins and 100 in individuals with varicose veins. Authors found that the prevalence of reflux might vary from 14% to 87% depending on the severity group of subjects. Of more relevance, reflux was detectable in all the segments of the saphenous and non saphenous veins, but the distal parts of the great saphenous vein (GSV) and its tributaries were the most frequently involved, with similar prevalence in the three groups of patients. In the overall 125 limbs with superficial vein incompetence, the below-knee segment of GSV was the most common site of reflux (68% of limbs) followed by the above-knee segment of GSV (55%), while the sapheno-femoral junction was involved in only 32% of cases. These findings supported that the involvement of terminal valve at the junctions as an obligatory starting point was not necessary for reflux to develop. Authors also found that in contralateral asymptomatic limbs of patients with clinically evident varicose veins the prevalence of reflux was relevant with higher frequency of distal reflux and limited involvement of saphenous-femoral junction (SFJ) and saphenous-popliteal junction (SPJ). In addition, multi-segmental reflux was also likely ranging from 18% to 95% of cases with higher prevalence in the group of patients with clinically relevant varicosities. Authors concluded that because the prevalence of distal reflux was comparable among the three groups, including asymptomatic limbs, distal location of the disease should represent the more initial and less severe stage of venous disorder. In early stages, there is a large prevalence of distal reflux and limited involvement of junctions. Other factors, such the extent, the severity, the time that the disease has been present, the rate of progression and the efficiency of calf muscle pump may be responsible for the development of sign and symptoms of venous insufficiency that will involve, in delayed stages, more proximal levels of the limb. Authors concluded that these findings could suggest an ascending or multifocal process of reflux in addition to or separate from a retrograde process.[14]

This assumption was confirmed by a further study of the same Authors specifically analyzing the progression of reflux [15] over 116 limbs of patients with chronic venous disease and delayed treatment who were longitudinally observed through at least 2 duplex ultrasound examinations. After a median of 19 months, Authors observed that clinical stage progression (in 11.2%) and anatomical extension (in 29%) had occurred. According to ultrasound pattern changes, anatomical extensions were observed both, in continuity with pre-existing reflux and as a new segment reflux. Indeed reflux was detected in 12.1% of limbs as a new segment reflux in new locations independent of the preexisting disease. Of relevance, reflux extensions detected in continuity with pre-existing incompetent sites occurred in 14.7% of limbs either in antegrade or retrograde fashion. This data contradicted the traditional assumption that primary reflux always develops starting at the SF junction from valve incompetence and proceeds in a retrograde matter. The Authors' findings indeed supported that the reflux could develop at one or different locations without junctional involvement, often affecting different veins that might not communicate with each other and can progress in retrograde or anterograde manner, and/or in both directions.[15]

Bernardini et al,[10] reported on longitudinal observations of venous patterns in patients with primary superficial venous disease who refused treatment and were followed with 6-month scheduled clinical and duplex ultrasound examinations. Localization, stage, and evolution of the venous patterns were compared. A total of 104 limbs in 99 patients were analyzed (12 males, 92 female; mean age 48.7 years). Presence of reflux was more frequent along great-saphenous vein and its tributaries (78/104, 75%) than non-saphenous veins. At the time of re-examination, ranging from 1 to 13 years (mean 4 ± 3.1 years), with the exception of six remaining stable, all the veins showed a progression of reflux and in 47 the disease involved deep circulation. In all the worsened refluxes, an extension to reach one or more venous segments at an upper level, uninvolved before, was found. There was no downward oriented pattern of progression. There was no significant difference in age, gender, and type of vein between the stable and progressive diseases. Despite the limited numbers, this experience further concluded about primary venous insufficiency as a progressive disease, which begins at lower levels of the limbs where venous stasis is higher, and develops in an antegrade manner.

Reflux and Perforator Veins

With the use of ultrasound mapping, the observation of patterns of nonsaphenous superficial refluxes where the terminal valves at the junctions were totally continents have becoming increasingly evident. [16]

A number of studies have recently shown indeed that venous reflux may occur because of high pressure entering in the superficial system through incompetent valves in perforator veins more than through SF valve incompetence at the SF junction. Perforator valve incompetence allows blood to flow from deep veins back into the superficial system and permits transmission of the high pressures generated by the calf muscle pump. This local high pressure can produce excessive vein dilatation and secondary failure of superficial vein valves. As a result, a cluster of dilated veins develops at this site (calf) and leads to ascending venous reflux.[16-18]

Moreover, Delis et al, observed that incompetent perforators in the lower third of the calf often have larger diameters than those in either the middle or upper calf thirds, these findings indicating that distal calf perforators may be of the most significance hemodinamically.[18]

To support this hypothesis, Labropoulos et al,[19] analyzed the longitudinal patterns of evolution of reflux (changes of detailed ultrasound maps) in the perforator veins in 158 limbs of patients with untreated primary venous disease and at least two examinations. Any new perforator vein reflux was anatomically recorded and classified in ascending type, descending type and those developed in new locations. The ascending development of reflux into perforating veins from previously competent segments of superficial veins was the more prevalent type of evolution involving 47.4% of limbs. In addition, a smaller number of incompetent perforators were detected in new locations that previously did not have reflux in any system. In these new sites, reflux development could have been either ascending or descending; however, in cases of "descending" involvement, perforator vein incompetence was always in continuity with a superficial vein connected to it, suggesting that more than a true descending (retrograde progression downwards to a distal level) evolution, the perforator incompetence represented the "re-entry point" of a superficial vein reflux located at the same level.

Hemodynamic principles have indeed suggested that reflux in the perforator veins may occur in the presence of incompetent superficial veins that act as a capacitor for the refluxing perforator. As the local hemodynamic conditions change and as intravenous pressure increases, the diameter of the perforator vein increases and the perforator valve becomes incompetent allowing reverse venous flow to decrease the hyper-pressurization in the superficial system. These re-entry flows through perforators are not always pathologic since they are not always supported by irreversible valve failure and are not associated with reflux in deep veins connected to them. Indeed, according to hemodynamic principles, the role of most perforators in determining varicose veins has been explained as a drainage escape in a "Private circulation" or "Shunt", that is an expression of a vicious circle of blood between the superficial and the deep circulations. The circle starts during muscular relaxation when the blood from the reflux point of the superficial veins flows to the re-entry point, represented by a perforating vein, and then into a deep vein. The circle ends during the following muscular contraction, when the blood flows forward through the deep veins and then again to the superficial reflux point when muscle relaxation occurs.[20]

Drainage perforating veins ("re-entry" points) are usually located at lower levels with respect to the connected superficial network capacitor of hyper-pressurized and varicose superficial veins. Perforators located at lower levels are indeed those receiving hyper-pressure and more prone to first dilate and allow a reverse flow. Nevertheless, this does not imply a downward, retrograde, progression of varicose disease but only shows that each superficial vein network has its escape re-entry point located distally where the pressure is higher. With the progression of the disease, the increase in pressure and venous stasis along perforator veins follows the pressure gradient: new perforators can become hyper-pressurized and can dilate at above levels not involved before with proximal extension of the disease. The disease therefore expands upwards involving new vein networks located above (superficial capacitors) with their related re-entry points (perforators).

Reflux and Tributaries Veins

Reflux has been also observed in venous tributaries in the absence of any axial or perforator reflux. Thus, reflux, confined to the superficial tributaries may occur throughout the limb, and importantly, the most common tributaries with reflux are easily located at the calf level and found in communication with the great saphenous vein (65%), the small saphenous vein (19%) or both (7%). [21-22] This process of isolated tributary reflux may contribute to progression of disease within the other venous segments with ascending evolution.

Labropoulos et al,[22] published about the observation of primary superficial vein reflux patterns without incompetence of the saphenous trunk. The study was based on longitudinal analysis of 84 limbs with symptoms of chronic venous disease in 62 patients and showed that reflux could be confined to superficial tributaries throughout the lower limb. The posterior arch tributaries veins of the calf were the most commonly involved and reflux was observed in below-the-knee tributaries alone (distal reflux) in 28% of limbs. Furthermore, multi-segmental incompetence was significantly more prevalent than segmental (80% vs 20%). Authors concluded that because the reflux is present along the lower limb without greater saphenous trunk, lesser saphenous trunk, perforator and deep-vein incompetence, it could develop in any vein without an apparent feeding source from an incompetent terminal valve. Again, the mandatory terminal valve starting point of primary varicose incompetence in lower limbs was not confirmed while a multifocal or ascending evolution of venous insufficiency was suggested.[22]

Similar occurrences of reflux were observed by Engelhorn et al.[23] who specifically analyzed ultrasound patterns of saphenous reflux in women with primary varicose veins. Ultrasound mapping was prospectively performed in 590 extremities of women with varicose veins and mild disease (CEAP C_2 class) without edema or ulcers. Distribution and patterns of Great saphenous vein (GSV), small saphenous vein (SSV) refluxes and non-saphenous refluxes were observed in upright position and recorded. Reflux was detected in 472 extremities with a 77% prevalence at the GSV and 20% at SSV level. Authors found that the most common pattern of reflux (58%) arose from a tributary or perforating vein to another tributary or perforating vein above the malleolar level and these refluxes were often multi-segmental (two or more distinct refluxing segments were detected). GSV refluxing segments were noted most commonly in the leg (distal type) or in the leg and thigh (58%) while involvement of thigh was present in 37% and of junction (SFJ) only in 12% of cases. Authors concluded that only about one third of CEAP C_2 limbs may require treatment of a refluxing saphenous vein in the thigh, supporting the ascending evolution of a disease that starts at the distal sites and in its minor stages (C_2) is confined in the distal leg. Only with advanced stages the varicose disease may progress to reach above the thigh and the junction.[23] These findings obviously applied to women population and prevented widespread generalization.

B. Clinical Data on Reflux with Competent Saphenous Junction

The ascending evolution theory became more likely from the increasing number of studies showing that saphenous reflux may occur without incompetence at the saphenous junction (Table II). It has been established that in cases of great saphenous vein reflux, the terminal junction valve is often continent and finding reflux in the groin does not imply that it originates at that point (saphenous junction). [13] The frequency of sub-junctional or more distal trunk reflux was evaluated around 50%.[11-16,24-27] Cappelli et al,[25] reported that approximately half the refluxes in the SF junctions presented with a competent terminal valve. [25]Wong et al, found junctional incompetence at 53% of primary saphenous-femoral junctions and incompetence at saphenous-popliteal junction in 42% of cases with popliteal reflux.[26] Presence of saphenous-femoral junction incompetence was associated with older age and more advanced and widespread varicose vein disease and multifocal reflux, these findings also suggesting the concept of an early treatment of venous insufficiency before predictable deterioration with involvement of junctions may occur.[27]

Table II. Clinical data on reflux with competent saphenous junctions

Authors	Year	Journal and title	Settings	Main findings	population
Abu Own et al,[11]	1994	*British Journal of Surgery* Saphenous vein reflux without incompetence at the saphenofemoral junction	Ultrasound examination of consecutive patients with primary varicose veins	63 great saphenous vein varicosities without junction incompetence	190
Labropoulos et al,[21]	2004	*European Journal of Vascular Endovascular Surgery* Sapheno-femoral junction reflux in patients with a normal saphenous trunk	Multicentric study on sapheno-femoral junction (SFJ) reflux in patients with chronic venous disease and normal great saphenous trunk	SFJ normal diameter: 21%, dilated: 62% and varicose: 17%. Prevalence of SFJ reflux: 6.9%	1500
Cooper et al,[28]	2003	*European Journal of Vascular Endovascular Surgery* Primary varicose veins: the saphenofemoral junction, distribution of varicosities and patterns of incompetence	Distribution of varicosity patterns in patients with primary varicose veins	46% competent SFJ. Varicosities most common in the calf (up to 82%). More widespread disease with SFJ incompetence	480
Barros et al,[29]	2006	*European Journal of Vascular Endovascular Surgery* Clinical significance of ostial great saphenous vein reflux	Anatomical and hemodynamic patterns by Duplex Ultrasound and air plethysmography	significant differences in saphenous vein diameter and plethysmography volumes with the higher values in the patients with incompetent junction	121
Caggiati et al,[30]	2006	*Journal of Vascular Surgery* Age-related variations of varicose veins anatomy	Age related varicose vein patterns	SFJ reflux in 38% young and in 59% elder. In most young varicose disease only on non saphenous veins (36%) or tributaries (25%)	338

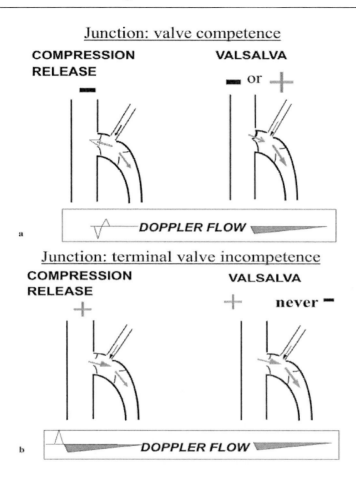

Figure 6. a. Junction levels: Valsalva positive or negative (right) while compression-release test is still negative (valve competence) (left). This represents initial stages of venous disease: saphenous junctions can dilate and are involved by incompetence under stress (Valsalva positive) but terminal valves are still competent under normal pressure conditions (Compression-test negative) . b. In advanced stages compression-release maneuvers will become positive in addition to the Valsalva, indicating that not only a functional dilation of the junction under hyper-pressure stimulation but a failure of the valve under normal pressure is occurred. The opposite, ie, positive compression-release test with negative Valsalva maneuver, never occurs.

The relationship between varicose vein and saphenous vein valves insufficiency has been studied from centuries. In examining saphenous junctions, different positive/negative results can be observed between compression-release test and Valsalva maneuver. The compression-release test reproduces the flow at the junction under normal conditions, while the

Valsalva provides a stress test where the junction is subjected to exaggerate pressure. There are limbs where both tests are negative because the junction is intact also under stress condition. However, there are also limbs in which negative compression-release test and positive Valsalva maneuver can be found, while the opposite, ie, positive compression-release test with negative Valsalva maneuver never occurs (Figure 6 a, b).

These findings support that at initial stages of venous incompetence the saphenous junctions can dilate and are involved by incompetence only under stress with high pressure (Valsalva positive) but terminal valves are still competent under normal pressure conditions (compression-test negative). Only in subsequent stages, compression maneuvers will become positive in addition to the Valsalva, indicating that, in more advanced diseases, not only a functional dilation of the junction under hyper-pressure stimulation but a failure of the valve under normal pressure is occurred. Indeed, with more advanced and severe disease vein dilatation will involve the vein wall at the junction widening the leaflets and finally allowing valve incompetence and reflux also under normal condition (compression-release test positive). Therefore, a persisting huge pressure is required to dilate and make incompetent the terminal saphenous-femoral valve at SF junction in previously incompetent veins with intact junctions. These findings can be again explained by the basic principles of the ascending theory: because of the increased hydrostatic pressure levels, the lowest limb level represents not only the starting point but also the point of more severe reflux responsible for developing the earliest symptoms and signs of venous insufficiency. The continuous increase in hydrostatic pressure will propagate upwards following the hydrostatic pressure gradient allowing progressive enlargement of the vein above that will finally involve the junction with, at first, only functional valve insufficiency under stress (Valsalva positive test). Finally, if not treated, the hyper-pressure will reach the terminal valve at junctions, allowing valve dilatation /failure with presence of persisting reflux under normal pressure and positive compression-release maneuvers.

Especially after the widespread use of ultrasound it has become a common finding that refluxes, even in the saphenous axis, are often found below competent terminal valves. Table II summarizes studies findings on this topic: in up to 67% of patients, saphenous reflux exists without SFJ (26.6%-67%) or saphenous-popliteal junction incompetence (42%). [10-16,24-28]

Already in the earlier nineties (1994), Abu Own et al,[11] suggested that in about one third of limbs with great saphenous vein reflux, there was no associated saphenous-femoral junction incompetence. After analyzing by ultrasound limbs in 167 consecutive patients with clinical diagnosis of primary varicose veins, Authors found that among 190 limbs with great saphenous vein incontinence, 63 had no SF junction incompetence. This was a clear demonstration that reflux along the saphenous trunk may often occur in the presence of a competent saphenous junction, suggesting that the development of primary varicose vein may be an ascending rather than retrograde phenomenon.

Labropoulos, Leon, Engelhorn et al, [21] specifically analyzed ultrasound patterns of varicosities in a large multicenter observational study of 1500 limbs in patients with evidence of chronic venous disease, to investigate the clinical importance of saphenous-femoral junction reflux. Assuming "7mm" as an ultrasound vein dilatation cut-off, Authors found that the junction had a normal diameter in 21%, was dilated in 62% and varicose in only 17% of limbs. Prevalence of SF junction reflux was 6.9%, and was seen in 39% of limbs with a normal junction diameter, in 85% of those with a dilated junction and in all varicose junctions. These findings indirectly supported that reflux was likely due to a local or multifocal process separate from a retrograde progression. Involvement of the junction was a late terminal stage in most cases.[21]

In 2003, Cooper et al,[28] retrospectively reviewed the duplex ultrasound patterns of venous duplex scan in 706 limbs of patients referred for treatment of primary varicose veins. They found that 46% of varicose limbs had a competent SF junction and varicosities were most commonly in the calf (up to 82%) occurring at or below the level of competences within the saphenous vein. Involvement of the thigh only was as low as 5.5% of cases, while the junction involvement was usually associated with more advanced and widespread disease (calf and thigh). Authors thereby concluded that it appeared unlikely that varicose veins developed from dysfunction of the valves of the superficial venous system in a descending fashion. More than starting from a single incompetent focal point located at the terminal valve in junction, varicose disease could develop at any position within the venous system. Furthermore, Authors suggested that more than an hyper-pressure involving terminal valve and superficial vein system from the deep veins, a more complex interaction between luminal forces and un-controlled molecular signals for venous vessels to dilate could be fundamental to the genesis and vein varicosities. The thought of a primary wall abnormality predisposing to venous dilatation as a precursor to later valve incompetence, and finally, reflux was therefore suggested as likely.[28]

The theory of a primary weakening of the venous wall as the initiating factor of reflux, has gained further support by the experience of Barros and Labroupulos in 2006,[29] based on hemodynamic and anatomical observations. Authors specifically investigated with Duplex Ultrasound and air plethysmography reflux distribution in 121 limbs of patients with (n=94) or without (n=27, control group) evidence of chronic venous disease. In 69 limbs a saphenous junction reflux was detected. There was a significant difference between the 2 groups in saphenous vein diameter evaluated by ultrasound and in total venous volume and venous filling index, evaluated by plethysmography, with the higher values in the group of patients with incompetent junction. Authors found that in patients with Great saphenous vein reflux, those with incompetence of the "ostial" (junction) valve had greater venous reflux and dilatation of the saphenous trunk than those in whom "ostial" valve was competent, thereby suggesting that the presence of a saphenous-femoral junction incompetence was not a prerequisite for varicose vein formation. Its presence more likely suggested a more advanced, late-staged disease with more severe hemodynamic compromise of veins; this indirectly supported the ascending progression of venous reflux.[29]

Caggiati et al, in 2006,[30] observed that distribution of venous incompetence can vary with age. Saphenous involvement and especially SF junction involvement is more common in older patients as an expression of a long-standing, more advanced, disease, while, in younger patients, varicosities, as an appearance of an earlier staged disease, are more likely located at distal leg along non-saphenous veins. Authors compared ultrasound patterns of 100 varicose limbs in younger patients (<30 years) and 238 limbs in older patients (>60years). Varicose saphenous veins were present in 62% of the older group and in 39% of the younger where most varicose changes affected only non-saphenous veins (36%) or saphenous tributaries (25%). Of relevance, the presence of junctional incompetence affected only 38% of young patients, while 59% of the elders showed incompetence of the junction. The frequent occurrence of normal saphenous trunk in varicose limbs (44%) allowed Authors to not support the crucial role commonly credited to the saphenous junction in the pathogenesis of primary varicosities, especially in young patients. Authors' findings more likely suggested that varicose disease might progressively extend in a centripetal fashion from distal tributaries veins into saphenous vein with an ascendent extension along the saphenous trunk up to the junction. These data confirmed that incompetence at the saphenous junctions associated with varicosities of the saphenous trunks made the disease more serious from the hemodynamic point of view and reflected a stage where the disease is more widespread rather than being the initiating factor/location.

C. Clinical Results after Varicose Vein Treatments with Preservation of Sapheno-Femoral Confluence (Junction Sparing)

The hypothesis of an ascending more than retrograde evolution of venous varicosities starting from the terminal valve received a noteworthy substantiation from studies showing the efficacy of varicose vein treatments with sparing the terminal valve and the saphenous junctions.

The suggestion of varicose incompetence as a disease process that originated at distal levels and regularly occurred in the absence of reflux at the SF junction raised the question as to whether an aggressive treatment of the saphenous junction was always justified. A number of studies indeed recently described the possibility of reflux elimination as the successful hemodynamic consequence of procedures performed without any direct action on the junctions (Table III). The shown efficacy of a variety of these approaches localized in the sub-junctional saphenous vein able also to recover terminal valve incompetence (without any direct action at the junctions level), is strictly dependent from the ascending progression of venous disease.

Pittaluga et al,[31] provided renewed interest to the treatment of varicose vein with the approach of "extensive varicose reservoir ablation" suggested by Muller et al,[32] long time ago in 1966, and extensively applied the technique of sparing the saphenous-femoral junction during surgical stripping of great saphenous vein in recent years. By reviewing the long-term postoperative outcome (>1 year) of 195 lower limbs treated for varicose saphenous vein with extensive varicose vein stripping but saphenous-femoral confluence preservation, Pittaluga et al. observed that persistent reflux at the confluence (neovascularization) was detected in only two cases after this treatment (1.8% at 2 years). Of relevance, the risk of thrombosis of the sapheno-femoral stump was also negligible (1 transient case).

After a mean of 24.4 months, 83.9% of limbs could be converted to less severe disease (CEAP clinical class 0 to 1) and significant symptoms improvement was observed in 91.3% of cases with an aesthetic benefit in 95.5%. Authors concluded that, due to hemodynamic consequences, the extensive ablation of saphenous varicose vein ("venous reservoir" ablation) might be even more beneficial without any treatment at the sapheno-femoral junction.

Table III. Clinical results after varicose vein treatments with preservation of saphenous-femoral confluence (Junction sparing)

Authors	Year	Journal and title	Settings	Main findings	Population
Pittaluga et al,[31]	2008	*Journal of Vascular Surgery* Great saphenous vein stripping with preservation of sapheno-femoral confluence: hemodynamic and clinical results	Retrospective analysis of outcomes after stripping of great saphenous with preservation of saphenous-femoral confluence (SFC)	At a mean of 24.4months: complete recovery 91.3%; persistent reflux 1.8%; SFC neovascularization 0.9%. One recurrence	195
Pittaluga et al,[33]	2009	*Journal of Vascular Surgery* Midterm results of the surgical treatment of varices by phlebectomy with conservation of a refluxing saphenous vein	Ambulatory selective varices ablation under local anesthesia (ASVAL) procedure	Ablation of varicose reservoir with conservation of a refluxing saphenous vein was effective treatment in >2/3 cases. Symptoms disappeared in 84.2% at 1 year and in 78.0% at 4 years Freedom from recurrences: 88.5% at 4 years	303
Bernardini et al,[35]	2007	*Annals of Vascular Surgery* Echosclerosis hemodynamic conservative: a new technique for varicose vein treatment	Echo-sclerosis hemodynamic conservative (ESEC) technique	junction incompetence reversal with sclerotherapy directed in the sub-junction saphenous vein trunk (ESEC 1) or in saphenous branches (ESEC 2)	980
Bernardini et al,[34]	2007	*Phlebologie* Ambulatoy and hemodynamic treatment of venous insufficiency by ultrasound-guided sclerotherapy: 14 year results	Early and long-term results after ESEC	Clinical/cosmetic improvement persisting after 14 years from ESEC. Mean vein diameter decrease in veins above the site of ESEC: 52%	146

The integrity of saphenous-femoral confluence during treatment of reflux in great saphenous vein could be worthwhile because of the preservation of inguinal venous drainage, while the extensive ablation of varicose vein reservoir (varicose superficial veins, mainly tributary) might allow the absence of an outflow for the reflux. Preserving the superficial abdominal and perineal venous drainage by not dissecting at all the saphenous-femoral confluence and by not dividing the collaterals at the junction, could indeed avoid neovascularization of the confluence while not preventing these collaterals from draining into the femoral vein. Thereby, saphenous stripping in association with extensive phlebectomies could improve hemodynamics of the preserved saphenous-femoral confluence, since the great saphenous vein cannot become permeable again.

The same Authors further found that venous reservoir ablation with preservation of saphenous-femoral confluence could be effective also in the presence of an already refluxing confluence. Furthermore, in less advanced diseases, ablative treatment could be successfully applied as a mini-invasive treatment by acting exclusively on tributary veins without any action on the saphenous trunk. Results were maintained in the mid-term (up to 4 years). Authors used mini-phlebectomies to obtain extensive ablation of varicosities (many were tributaries and collaterals) with the conservation of a preoperatively refluxing saphenous vein, the so called Ambulatory Selective Varices Ablation under Local Anesthesia (ASVAL). ASVAL was applied in 303 limbs with saphenous reflux. Post-operative and midterm outcomes were compared with 270 limbs treated with high ligation associated with stripping.[33] After ASVAL, reflux could be reduced in 69% limbs after 6 months and in 66.3% of limbs after 4 years of follow-up. Symptoms improved or disappeared in more than 80% of limbs at 4 years. The demonstrated efficacy in treatment in two of three cases of saphenous reflux with ASVAL could be only explained whether an ascending development of varicose disease starting from the distal superficial venous network was accepted: venous incompetence followed an ascending progression from the collaterals to the saphenous veins leading the ASVAL treatment to reverse saphenous reflux after removing the varicose reservoir even when no direct action on the saphenous junction was used. Authors concluded that using mini-invasive technique, surgical ablation of varicose reservoir with conservation of a refluxing sapheno-femoral junction could be an effective treatment in the midterm and could be competitive with other mini-invasive approaches such as endovenous ablation.[33]

Other mini-invasive techniques with sparing of the saphenous-femoral junction but also with conservative and selective varicose vein treatment (at the opposite of the extensive reservoir ablation used in the ASVAL) were also successfully applied to support the ascending theory. This was achieved by sclerotherapy with the so called Echo-Sclerosis haEmodynamic Conservative (ESEC),[34] a new treatment method for sclerotherapy conceived to achieve venous stasis suppression by following hemodynamic approach that preserves venous drainage vessels and saphenous-femoral junctions. The objective was obtained through a super-selective, ultrasound-guided sclerosis, specifically directed into a saphenous segment (ESEC 1 technique) or into a saphenous branch (ESEC 2 technique or indirect technique) over a confluence point through which drainage into deep circulation could be directed. Authors based their technique on hemodynamic concepts of venous disease: the selective interruption of the hydrostatic pressure column along the venous axis with sclerotherapy localized at the reflux sites (either branches or saphenous trunk) might allow to decrease the pressure weight on the veins below, since the height of the hydrostatic column is shortened (the breakage splits the single longer hydrostatic column in two shorter columns, each with a lower weight). At the same time, after such interruption, venous flow will be likely redirected through collateral branches or perforating veins (namely, "reentry perforating veins") in a physiologic one-way ("superficial to deep") pattern. These recovered re-entries flows can allow an efficient venous drainage of the above varicose segments previously hyper-pressurized since overflowed from the reflux point (now interrupted). These hemodynamic corrected and physiologically redirected, low-pressure flows can therefore permit depressurization and shrinkage of the upward superficial varicose segment/ networks up to the above valve that will recover continence ("segmental venous insufficiency recover"). In the same way the terminal valve at the SFJ may be also recovered once the sub-junctional saphenous vein shrink after the sclerotherapy interruption of the weight pressure at a level below. If hemodynamic abnormalities are not corrected by breaking the pressure column, the increase of hydrostatic pressure within the varicose veins with the time will get worse and will propagate upward (following the longitudinal hydrostatic pressure gradient) causing progressive vein dilatation, valve detachment with incompetence and development of reflux into the above venous axis.

The ESEC Authors reviewed their approach to treat 146 varicose veins and found that with this superconservative technique of sclerotherapy the saphenous trunk integrity could be preserved and the terminal valve competence reestablished without any direct treatment of SJ.[35] Indeed, in 90.6% of patients the terminal valve continence was restored after selective sclerosis in selected lower venous segments either within or outside the saphenous trunk. Furthermore, the mean venous diameter in the veins above the site of ESEC application decreased of about 50% after the procedure applied below. The efficacy of treatment was found to persist after 14years.[34]

Of relevance, the ascending theory was supported by two totally different junction sparing approaches to venous disease as the AVAL and the ESEC. Even with different basic concepts both the techniques showed the efficacy after preserving the sapheno-femoral junction and raised doubts against the benefit of extensive junction treatments. The ASVAL was essentially based on the concept to exclude all reflux points by extensive ablation of all the superficial varicose veins (venous reservoir, mainly consisting of tributaries veins) while preserving the saphenous-femoral confluence (and most of the saphenous vein) to allow drainage from collaterals into the femoral vein (deep circulation). The ESEC was a more conservative technique that was based on the principle of breaking by sclerotherapy the hydrostatic column of venous pressure along the leg. The decrease of venous pressure allowed the shrinkage of the venous segments above the point of selective sclerosis, with recovery of normal size and valve competence. The sclerosis was always applied below the junction level using a superselectively approach in a target vein above a confluence point to allow venous flow drainage into deep circulation and thereby decrease the pressure column. With the shrinkage of the junctional segment, junctional valve incompetence could be restored without any application of therapy on the junction.

CONCLUSION

In conclusion, increasing evidence is suggesting that the development of primary venous insufficiency can follow an ascending pattern where the terminal valve is the last to be involved. This is conflicting with the traditional "retrograde" theory stating that the incompetence of valves above the saphenous-femoral junction is the primary source of varicose disease that proceeds in a retrograde manner with progressive dilatation and valve incompetence downwards the saphenous vein and its tributaries. Nevertheless, the pathophysiologic mechanisms that lead to the development and progression of vein reflux in lower limbs have not found uniform consensus and the retrograde theory of reflux still remains largely accepted.

The ascending evolution is supported by hemodynamic principles, literature data and direct observations that can be summarized as follows:

1. According to scientific laws, the development of venous insufficiency in lower limb is likely determined by the hydrostatic column of venous pressure and thereby follows the gravity gradient along the column. The lower the level (higher the gravity force), the higher the hydrostatic pressure causing venous incompetence and the reflux to begin. Once started a lower point, varicose vein disease can subsequently evolve uprising in accordance with the pressure gradient.

2. There is evidence to support that terminal valve involvement in varicose disease of saphenous vein can occur in less half population with venous insufficiency. In 45-55% of cases refluxes along saphenous vein are found below competent terminal valves that are therefore last components to be involved from venous insufficiency.

3. Studies using selective and minimally invasive approach to treat varicose veins have shown that after treatment localized in a target vein, the shrinkage and recovery of the of dilated varicose vein above can occur. This might not be explained with a retrograde development of varicose disease where the disease at above levels should be antecedent and prelude the involvement of lower venous segments.

The natural history of varicose veins is that of a progressive disease which chronic evolution. Although the exact development is uncertain, it is likely that the disease begins at the lower levels of the limbs and develops in an antegrade manner as venous stasis is higher where force of gravity is higher. This data might be of relevance in planning treatment since do not support an aggressive and widespread treatment of the terminal valve as first strategy in the presence of varicose veins of lower limbs.

REFERENCES

[1]   Beebe-Dimmer JL, Pfeifer JR, Engle JS, et al: The epidemiology of chronic venous insufficiency and varicose veins. *Ann. Epidemiol.* 2005; 15:175-184.

[2]   Callam MJ. Epidemiology of varicose veins. *Br. J. Surg.* 1994;81:167-73. Review.

[3]   Criqui MH, Jamosmos M, Fronek A, et al: Chronic venous disease in an ethnically diverse population: the San Diego Population Study. *Am. J. Epidemiol.* 2003; 158:448-456.

[4]   Evans CJ, Fowkes FG, Ruckley CV, et al: Prevalence of varicose veins and chronic venous insufficiency in men and women in the general population: Edinburgh Vein Study. *J. Epidemiol. Community Health* 1999; 53:149-153.

[5]   Ludbrook J, Beale G. Femoral venous valves in relation to varicose veins. *Lancet* 1962;1:79-81.

[6]   Lurie F. Venous haemodynamics: what we know and don't know. *Phlebology.* 2009;24:3-7.

[7]   Pascarella L, Schmid Schonbein GW. Causes of telangiectasias, reticular veins and varicose veins. *Semin. Vasc. Surg* 2005;18:2-4.

[8]   Venruri M, Bonavina L, Annoni F, Colombo L, Butera C, Perachia A. Biochemical assay of collagen and elastin in the normal and varicose vein wall. *J. Surg. Res.* 1996;60: 245-248.

[9]   Travers JP, Brookes CE, Evans J, et al. Assessment of wall structure and composition of varicose veins with reference to collagen, elastin and smooth muscle cell content. *Eur. J. Vasc. Endovasc. Surg.* 1996;11:230-237.

[10] Bernardini E, De Rango P, Piccioli R, Bisacci C, Pagliuca V, Genovese G, Bisacci R. Development of primary superficial venous insufficiency: the ascending theory. Observational and hemodynamic data from a 9-year experience. *Ann. Vasc. Surg.* 2010;24:709-20.

[11] Abu-Own A, Scurr JH, Coleridge Smith PD. Saphenous vein reflux without incompetence at the saphenofemoral junction. *Br. J. Surg.* 1994;81:1452-1454.

[12] Perrin MR, Labropoulos N, Leon LR, Jr. Presentation of the patient with recurrent varices after surgery (REVAS). *J. Vasc. Surg.* 2006;43:327-334.

[13] García-Gimeno M, Rodríguez-Camarero S, Tagarro-Villalba S, Ramalle-Gomara E, González-González E, Arranz MA, García DL, Puerta CV. Duplex mapping of 2036 primary varicose veins. *J. Vasc. Surg.* 2009 Mar;49(3):681-9.

[14] Labropoulos N, Giannoukas AD, Delis K, Mansour MA, Kang SS, Nicolaides AN, Lumley J, Baker WH. Where does venous reflux start? *J. Vasc. Surg.* 1997 Nov;26(5):736-42.

[15] Labropoulos N, Leon L, Kwon S, Tassiopoulos A, Gonzalez-Fajardo JA, Kang SS, et al. Study of the venous reflux progression. *J. Vasc. Surg.* 2005;41:291-5.

[16] Labropoulos N, Tiongson J, Pryor L, Tassiopoulos AK, Kang SS, Mansour MA, Baker WH. Nonsaphenous superficial vein reflux. *J. Vasc. Surg.* 2001 Nov;34(5):872-7.

[17] Labropoulos N, Mansour MA, Kang SS, et al: New insight into perforator vein incompetence.. *Euro. J. Vasc. Surg.* 1999; 18:228-234.

[18] Delis KT, Husmann M, Kalodiki E, et al: In situ hemodynamics or perforating veins in chronic venous insufficiency. *J. Vasc. Surg.* 2001; 33:773-782.

[19] Labropoulos N, Tassiopoulos AK, Bhatti AF, Leon L. Development of reflux in the perforator veins in limbs with primary venous disease. *J. Vasc. Surg.* 2006 Mar;43(3):558-62.

[20] Carandina S, Mari C, De Palma M, Marcellino MG, Cisno C, Legnaro A, Liboni A, Zamboni P. Varicose vein stripping vs haemodynamic correction (CHIVA): a long term randomised trial. *Eur. J. Vasc. Endovasc. Surg.* 2008 Feb;35(2):230-7.

[21] Labropoulos N, Leon L, Engelhorn CA, Amaral SI, Rodriguez H, Kang SS, Mansour AM, Littooy FN. Sapheno-femoral junction reflux in patients with a normal saphenous trunk. *Eur. J. Vasc. Endovasc. Surg.* 2004 Dec;28(6):595-9.

[22] Labropoulos N, Kang SS, Mansour MA, Giannoukas AD, Buckman J, Baker WH. Primary superficial vein reflux with competent saphenous trunk. *Eur. J. Vasc. Endovasc. Surg.* 1999 Sep;18(3):201-6.

[23] Engelhorn CA, Engelhorn AL, Cassou MF, Salles-Cunha SX. Patterns of saphenous reflux in women with primary varicose veins. *J. Vasc. Surg.* 2005 Apr;41(4):645-51.

[24] Labropoulos N, Delis K, Nicolaides AN, Leon M, Ramaswami G. The role of the distribution and anatomic extent of reflux in the development of signs and symptoms in chronic venous insufficiency. *J. Vasc. Surg.* 1996;23:504-10.

[25] Cappelli M, Molino Lova R, Ermini S, Zamboni P. Hemodynamics of the sapheno-femoral junction. Patterns of reflux and their clinical implications. *Int. Angiol.* 2004 Mar;23(1):25-8.

[26] Wong JK, Duncan JL, Nichols DM. Whole-leg duplex mapping for varicose veins: observations on patterns of reflux in recurrent and primary legs, with clinical correlation. *Eur. J. Vasc. Endovasc. Surg.* 2003 Mar;25(3):267-75.

[27] Pittaluga P, Chastane S, Rea B, Barbe R. Classification of saphenous refluxes: implications for treatment. *Phlebology.* 2008;23(1):2-9.

[28] Cooper DG, Hillman-Cooper CS, Barker SG, Hollingsworth SJ. Primary varicose veins: the saphenofemoral junction, distribution of varicosities and patterns of incompetence. *Eur. J. Vasc. Endovasc. Surg.* 2003;25:53-59.

[29] Barros MV, Labropoulos N, Ribeiro AL, Okawa RY, Machado FS. Clinical significance of ostial great saphenous vein reflux. *Eur. J. Vasc. Endovasc. Surg.* 2006 Mar;31(3):320-4.

[30] Caggiati A, Rosi C, Heyn R, Franceschini M, Acconcia MC. Age-related variations of varicose veins anatomy. *J. Vasc. Surg.* 2006 Dec;44(6):1291-5.

[31] Pittaluga P, Chastanet S, Guex JJ. Great saphenous vein stripping with preservation of sapheno-femoral confluence: hemodynamic and clinical results. *J. Vasc. Surg.* 2008 Jun;47(6):1300-4.

[32] Muller R. Traitement des varices par phlébectomie ambulatoire. *Phlébologie* 1966;19:277-9.

[33] Pittaluga P, Chastanet S, Rea B, Barbe R. Midterm results of the surgical treatment of varices by phlebectomy with conservation of a refluxing saphenous vein. *J. Vasc. Surg.* 2009 Jul;50(1):107-18.

[34] Bernardini E, Piccioli R, De Rango P, Bisacci C, Pagliuca V, Bisacci R. Ambulatory and hemodynamic treatment of venous insufficiency by ultrasound-guided sclerotherapy: 14 year results. *Phlebologie* 2007;4:186-195.

[35] Bernardini E, Piccioli R, De Rango P, Bisacci C, Pagliuca V, Bisacci R. Echo-sclerosis hemodynamic conservative: a new technique for varicose vein treatment. *Ann. Vasc. Surg.* 2007 Jul;21(4):535-43.

In: Varicose Veins   ISBN 978-1-61209-841-8
Editor: Andrea L. Nelson   ©2011 Nova Science Publishers, Inc.

Chapter 4

TREATMENT OF VARICOSE VEINS BY ULTRASOUND-GUIDED FOAM SCLEROTHERAPY

Takashi Yamaki[1]

Department of Plastic and Reconstructive Surgery, Tokyo Women's
Medical University, Tokyo, Japan

ABSTRACT

After the introduction of foam form of sclerosing solution, foam
sclerotherapy rapidly gained its popularity. Nowadays, variety of venous
disorder can be treated with foam sclerotherapy with low rate of adverse
events. This Chapter presents the efficacy and safety of ultrasound-guided
foam sclerotherapy for varicose veins and updates previous publications.

INTRODUCTION

The first attempt at intravenous injection of a substance into the human
body dates back to Sigismund Elsholz (1623-1688),[1] who injected distilled

---

[1]Correspondence to: Takashi Yamaki M.D. Department of Plastic and Reconstructive Surgery,
Tokyo Women's Medical University, 8-1, Kawada-cho, Shinjuku-ku, Tokyo, 162-8666,
JAPAN. TEL: +81-3-3353-8111. FAX: +81-3-3225-0940. E-mail: yamaki@prs.twmu.ac.jp
Yamakit@aol.com .

plantain water into a branch of the crural vein to irrigate a venous ulcer. The first attempt at true "sclerotherapy" was made in 1682 by Zollikofer, who injected an acid into a vein to induce an intravenous thrombus.[1] Using animals, Pravaz performed intravascular injection of absolute ethanol to create thrombi in arterial malformations. He then used ferric chloride for treatment of varicose veins. In the early part of the 20th Century, many different compounds were tested as sclerosing solutions, including 50% grape sugar, mercury biiodiode, 20% and 30% sodium salicylate, sodium citrate, 20% to 30% sodium chloride, 1% bichloride of mercury, 50% to 60% calorose, 12% quinine sulfate with 6% urethane. These solutions were subsequently abandoned because of unacceptable levels of allergic reactions, necrosis and even fatalities.[2]

The modern day treatment of varicose veins using new agents that were classified as detergent sclerosing agents, began in 1930, when sodium morrhuate was first used by Higgins and Kittel. Ethanolamine oleate was used for the first time in 1937 by Biegeleisen. One of the most commonly used detergents today, sodium tetradecyl sulfate (STS), was first applied by Reiner in 1946. The use of polidocanol, recognized as another very commonly employed sclerosing agent, was reported by Henschel and Eichenberg in 1966. The importance of compression therapy, which was performed by Hippocrates as long ago as the fourth century BC, was re-emphasized by Sigg,[3] Orbach, [4] and Fegan,[5] in combination with modern sclerosing techniques.

HISTORY OF FOAM SCLEROTHERAPY

Historically, McAusland was the first to propose the use of "froth" for treatment of telangiectasia. His technique for obtaining foam was simply shaking a rubber-capped bottle filled with sodium morrhuate, and the froth was aspirated into a syringe.[6] In 1944, Orbach reported the air-block method,[7] which he used only for smaller and medium-sized varicose veins. For larger veins he recommended the conventional technique, without air-block. In 1949, Karl Sigg applied the air-block technique for larger veins, and reported more than 4,000 treatments performed without complications.[8] In 1950, Orbach re-introduced his air-block technique, which allowed him to improve the success rate by 10%.[9] Using his technique, however, only 20% of the sclerosant was transformed into foam with bubbles of relatively large and irregular caliber, and the side effects caused by this method led to its abandonment. Therefore, foam sclerotherapy did not become widely useduntil the mid 1990s after the introduction of new methods for transforming sclerosing solutions.

Several different methods for the production of various foam forms have been reported. In 1995, Cabrera proposed the injection of a physiologic gas (CO_2) into a detergent sclerosing agent,[10]and in 1997 he presented the results of sclerotherapy over a period of 5 years using micro-bubble foam prepared in this way.[11] In 1997, Monfreux described an "on-site" production technique that generated a simple foam with air in a glass syringe,[12]and later Henriet reported his experience using Monfreux's technique for minor varices.[13]He maintained that the foam differed from that produced by Orbach in terms of regularity, stability and durability. In 1998, Benigni and Sadoun proposed mixing the sclerosing agent with air in a disposable plastic syringe.[14]They reported a study comparing the short-term efficacy of 0.25% polidocanol foam with a liquid foam for the treatment of telangiectases. [15]Mingo-Garcia developed a special device for producing a foam using compressed air.[16]In 2000, Tessari reported a new method for the production of foam with two syringes connected with a three-way stopcock, which was later named the "Tessari method". His Italian colleagues rapidly adopted this technique, and it has been widely accepted for producing a stable foam.[17] In 2000, Sica and Benigni reported their 3-years experience with duplex-guided sclerotherapy for saphenous trunks using tetradecyl sulfate, and demonstrated the advantages of the foam in comparison with liquid form.[18]Similarly in 2000, Frullini and Cavezzi described their experience with duplex-guided foam sclerotherapy and evaluated its effects and safety.[19]

PRODUCTION OF SCLEROSANT FOAM

Three methods are recommended for preparation of stable foam according to the First European Consensus Meeting on Foam Sclerotherapy (ECMFS).[20]Monfreux described a method requiring a glass syringe, which producedsmall quantities of POL foam, and he used this in aseries of patients with truncal varicose veins.[13]Monfreux generated an absolutenegative pressure by placing a cap on the syringe.Although all concentrations of sclerosants can be usedwith this method, the optimal ratio of gas andsclerosant and the ideal bubble size have not yet been defined.[16] Sclerosing foam can be easily produced by Tessari's method using two syringes and a three-way stopcock. Basically, 1% and 3% POL are used.A 5-ml syringe is filled with

0.5 ml of POL, and 2.0 ml of air is aspirated with another 5-ml syringe. The two syringes are attached by a three-way stopcock, and stable sclerosing foam is obtained by mixing them through multiple passages between the two syringes (Figure 1).

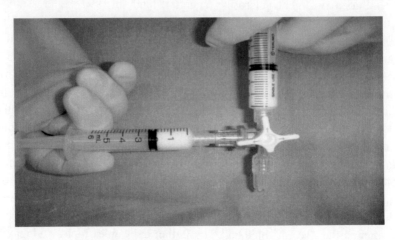

Figure 1.Tessari method for producing sclerosant foam.

However, foams can differ in consistency and show non-homogeneous flow behavior if minor changes are made during preparation. In laboratory experimental studies, efforts have been made to find the best possible combinations of connector type, syringe size, liquid-to-gas ratio, sclerosant concentration and manufacturing instructions. This has resulted in what is known as the "double-syringe system" (DSS) or "Tessari/DSS."[22, 23] Tessari/DSS foam, basedon the basic method devised by Tessari, is generated withtwo disposable silicone- and latex-free 10-ml plasticsyringes (one with a rubber plunger). One syringecontains 1 part liquid sclerosant, the other contains 4 parts gas. The outlets of the syringes (preferably Luer-Lock) are linked by a two-way connector at a 180°angle. The contents of the two syringes are pumped backwards and forwards 5 times(generating additional pressure by firmly holding the plunger of one syringe) and then again 7 times (withoutadditional pressure).[24]

At the Second ECMFS, the Tessari method and the Tessari/DSS were recommended for all indications. Only a few experts use Monfreux's technique for reticular and telangiectatic veins.[24] The preferred liquid:gas ratio for a foam sclerosant is 1:4.Ratios of between 1:1and 1:5 areusedfor reticular varicose veinsandspider veins, butthe 1:4 ratio is employed in the majority of cases.

PATIENT SELECTION

Generally, patients with primary valvular insufficiency showing reflux in the superficial and perforating veins are good candidates for foam sclerotherapy. It can be carriedout successfully in almost all patients with clinicallysignificant venous disease,irrespective of whether they are elderly, frail, obese or ill.[25]In principal, veins of all calibers with primary valvular insufficiency and recurrent varicose veins are suitable for foam sclerotherapy. To obtain better results, the larger the diameter of the vein, the more viscous the foam should be. A lower diameter threshold exists for viscous foams, whereas an upper diameter threshold is recognized for liquid forms, although no lower caliber limit has been defined.

Compression sclerotherapy is best performed on an ambulatory basis. Therefore, at the First ECMFS,sclerotherapy was not considered appropriate for patients who need to travel a long-distance and who require bedrest. Patients with a known allergic reaction to the sclerosant and a history of deep vein thrombosis and/or pulmonary embolism should not receive sclerotherapy. Patients who are known to have thrombophilia, a family history of thromboembolism, or severe arterial insufficiency of the limbs (stage 3 or 4) are also excluded from any treatment using sclerosing solutions. Sclerotherapy is absolutely contraindicated for patients who have systemic disease or hyperthyroidism.[20] The useof restricted amounts of foam is recommended for patients with symptomatic patent foramen ovale (PFO). However, at the Second ECMFS, symptomaticPFO wasconsidered anabsolutecontraindication for foam sclerotherapy. In addition, foam sclerotherapy is contraindicated for known asymptomatic PFO, although it is not considered necessary to check forPFO before foam sclerotherapy.[24]

DIAGNOSTICS BEFORE SCLEROTHERAPY

Proper evaluation of patients is the key for obtaining successful results of sclerotherapy. The diagnostic work-up includes a study of the patient's medical history, clinical examinations, and Doppler ultrasonography. Currently, duplex scanning is considered to be an important front-line test for patients with primary valvular insufficiency. Duplex scanning can detect the distribution as well as the extent of venous reflux. Although patients with primary valvular insufficiency may have various distributions of superficial, deep and perforating vein reflux, over90% of them have superficial venousinsufficiency with or without deep and perforating vein incompetence (Figure 2A, 2B).[27] Even in patients with combinedsuperficial and deep vein insufficiency, ablationof reflux in the superficial venous systemmay lead to resolution of deep vein reflux.[28, 29]Therefore, foam sclerotherapy is agood treatment option for such patients.

a)

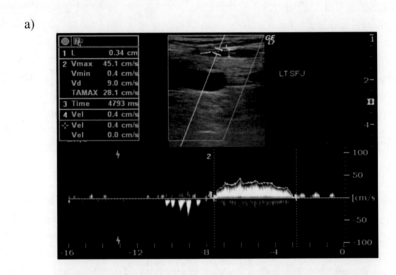

b)

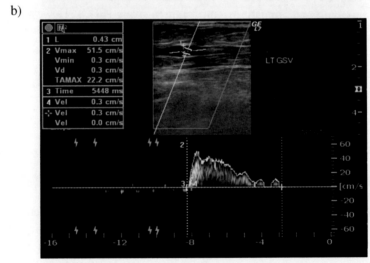

Figure 2. Evaluation of venous reflux at the sapheno-femoral junction (2A) and in the great saphenous vein (2B).

Additionally, functional testing can detect improvement of venous function. Recent studies have shown that air plethysmography (APG) can provide quantitative measurements of venous reflux, and that the amount of reflux is closely related to disease severity.[30, 31] Combined use of non-invasive diagnostic testing is also useful for follow-up of patients after sclerotherapy.

DUPLEX ULTRASOUND-GUIDED SCLEROTHERAPY

Theoretically, ultrasound-guided sclerotherapy should improve the results of treatment for a refluxing great saphenous vein (GSV). Using duplex ultrasound guidance, safe injections can be carried out by an experienced sclerotherapist.[32,33] Bishop and associates reported a GSV obliteration rate of only 6% when treating reflux without duplex guidance.[34] In contrast, Kanter and associates reported recanalization rates of 24.1% at 1 year and 35.7% at 2 years using duplex-guided sclerotherapy, which thus appears to be superior to conventional sclerotherapy.[35]At the moment, a wide range of different practices are employed for sclerotherapy.

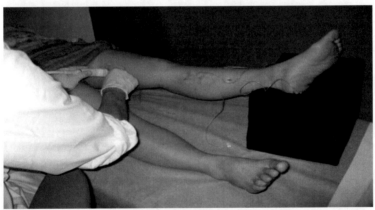

Note: butterfly needles are inserted into varicose tributary veins.

Figure 3. Ultrasound-guided polidocanol-foam sclerotherapy of the great saphenous vein.

In the Consensus Conference on Sclerotherapy held at Padua in 1994-1995, ultrasound-guided sclerotherapy was recommended for small saphenous varicose veins, anterior saphenous varicose veins, recurrent varicose veins, perforators, and obese patients.[36] No agreement was reached regarding the need for ultrasound-guided sclerotherapy, or the advantages of this treatment, for GSV incompetence.[36] At the First and Second ECMFS, however, duplex guidance was recommended, because it can help to confirm the intravenous placement of needles, catheter tips or any other means of vein access (Figure 3). [20, 24] Furthermore, duplex scanning allows easy identification of foam, and the initial effects are visible in real time (Figure4). It can also demonstrate whether large amounts offoamreach regions beyond the intended field of treatment.

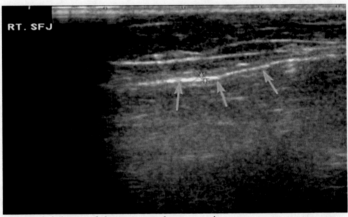

Note: complete shrinkage of the great saphenous vein.

Figure 4. Duplex scanning showing the injection of foam (arrows).

RECENT RANDOMIZED CONTROLLED TRIALS OF SCLEROSANT FOAM AND LIQUID FOR GSV REFLUX

The results of recent randomized controlled trials(RCTs) have shown a significantly higher response rate for sclerosant foamthan for liquid foam in the treatment of GSV incompetence. The response rateshave differed greatly among studycenters, as shown in Table 1. Some ofthese published RCTs were conducted at a single center, some used significantly greater foam volumes, sometimessmaller GSVs were treated, or tributaries wereinjected during the same session.[37-40]The efficacy rates for liquid foam were only 12% to 40% after periods of between 3 weeks and 2 years. The efficacy rates for sclerosant foam ranged from 53% to 84% during same follow-up period.If previous sclerotherapy has not completely occludedthevein orrecanalizationhas occurred, successful results can be obtained if further injections are performed (Figure 5). [41].

Table1. Results of recent controlled trials of liquid and foam

	Injected volume	No. of patients (POL-L and POL-F)	Efficacy criteria	Efficacy rate (POL-L and POL-F)
Hamel-Desnos C et al. [37] 2003	2.0-2.5 mL 3% POL-L or 3% POL-F	43 (POL-L) 45 (POL-F)	3 weeks after one treatment session: elimination of reflux	40% (POL-L) 84% (POL-F)
Yamaki T et al. [38] 2004	2 mL of 1% POL-L or POL-F for each draining vein into the GSV 2 mL of 3% POL-L or POL-F for GSV	40 (POL-L) 37 (POL-F)	12 months after one treatment session: complete occlusion of the GSV	17.5% (POL-L) 67.6% (POL-F)
Rabe E et al. [39] 2008	3.8 mL POL-F	52 (POL-L) 54 (POL-F)	3 months after last injection: elimination of reflux 3 cm below the SFJ	17% (POL-L) 54% (POL-F)
Ouvry P et al. [40] 2008	2.0-2.5 mL 3% POL-L or 3% POL-F	48 (POL-L) 47 (POL-F)	2 years after treatment: no recanalization	12% (POL-L) 53% (POL-F)

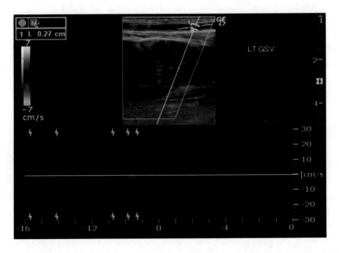

Figure 5. Post-sclerotherapy duplex scanning, showing complete occlusion of the above-knee great saphenous vein.

COMPARISON OF ULTRASOUND-GUIDED FOAM SCLEROTHERAPY WITH OTHER TREATMENT OPTIONS

There have beenonly two large randomizedcontrolled studies comparing foam sclerotherapy with other treatment options. [42, 43] Wright et al. performed an open-label, multicenter, prospective trial of 710 patients randomized to receiveeither Varisolve® or an alternative treatment (surgery or sclerotherapy).Overall, Varisolve® was shown to have non-inferiority with an efficacy of 83.4%, compared with 88.1% for alternative treatment at three months, and the corresponding rates at 12 months were 78.9% and 80.4%, respectively. Varisolve®was superior to sclerotherapy at 12 months. [42]Bountouroglou et al. compared ultrasound-guided foam sclerotherapy combined with sapheno-femoral ligation andsurgical treatment of varicose veins from a socio-economic viewpoint, and found that the former was less expensive and allowed more rapid recovery. [43]

With regard to recent endovenous treatment methods employing foam sclerotherapy, a non-randomized prospective study comparing foam sclerotherapy and endovenous laser ablation (EVLA) for GSV reflux reported cumulative occlusion rates at one year of 93% for EVLA and 77% for foam, as determined by ultrasound.[44] Furthermore, a systematic review of studies on theeffectiveness of four different therapies – foam sclerotherapy, surgical stripping, EVLA and radiofrequency ablation (RFA) – demonstrated a saphenous obliteration rate of 78% for surgical stripping, 77% for foam sclerotherapy,84% for RFA, and 94% for EVLA, after a meanfollow-up of 32 months.[45] Thus, the minimally invasive techniques appeared to be at least as effective as surgery for the treatment of lower extremity varicose veins.

SAFETY ASPECTS OF FOAM SCLEROTHERAPY

Because of its efficacy and safety, ultrasound-guided foam sclerotherapy has gained great popularity as a minimally invasive treatment for varicose veins, and large case series have been reported. Foam sclerosants can displace blood and adhere better to the walls of veins. However, recent reports have focused attention on the safety of foam for this purpose. Complications associated with foam sclerotherapy are generally uncommon. In a multicenterregistry of 12,173 sessions,the prevalence of complications associated with liquid sclerotherapy was 0.22% persession,and that of foam sclerotherapy was 0.58%.[46] In comparison with liquid sclerosant, foam sclerosant shows a greater tendency to provoke inflammation, and is consequently associated with mild adverse effects including pain, inflammatory signs, and skin pigmentation.[47] Furthermore, neurologic complications including transient visual disturbance, transient confusion, and even cerebral infarction have been described.[46-49]

GAS MIXTURE

The gas mixture used to create the bubbles in foam may be a factor that can provoke air embolism. Air has been commonly employed, but a more physiological gas might have certain advantages. Bubble life is shorter if the O_2 concentration within the bubble is higher and the nitrogen concentration lower.[50] Bubblesare much smaller when $CO_2$is used, and are more stable when amixture of CO_2 and O_2 is employed. Morrison et al. compared the incidence of side effects between carbon dioxide foam and air-based foam.[51] Concerning dizziness, they found a significant incidence of 12% when air-based foam was used, decreasing to 3% with CO_2-based foam. Overall, the proportion of patients describing side effects decreased from 39% to 11% as CO_2 replaced air for foam preparation ($p<0.001$).

FOAM CONCENTRATION AND VOLUME

The injected volume of sclerosant foam could also affect the incidence of side effects. The concentration of sclerosing solutions depends largely on the location of veins and vein diameter. The preferred foamvolumes per venous puncture are shown in Table 2,and the preferred concentrations are outlined inTable 3.[24]At the SecondECMFS, a statement was issued recommending 10 ml per session,[24]but different published reports have cited volumes ranging from 3 ml up to 30 ml. A case of stroke was reportedly associated with ultrasound-guided foam sclerotherapy for GSV incompetence employing 20 ml of POL-foam prepared by the Tessari method.[49] Theoretically, an air embolism can be fatal if a volume of >1 ml/kg is entrained into the venous system, but problems can also occur with a volume as small as 50 ml.[48] At lower foam doses, the total gas load of the bubbles is better solubilized, and the bubbles may become well separated spatially, reducing coalescence. [50]Deep vein thromboses have been reported with large (20 ml)[52] of very large amounts (33 ml and more) [53] of foam.However, another report has stated that there is no available evidence to suggest that larger volumes areassociated with any increased risk to patients receiving ultrasound-guided foam sclerotherapy.[54] A recent study has shown that multiple injections of <0.5 ml 1% POL-Frather than a few injections of >0.5 ml 1% POL-F per injection can reduce the amount of foam sclerosant and the risk of the sclerosant entering the deep veins in patients with superficial venous insufficiency. [55]

Table 2. Preferred foam volume per puncture
(From Breu FX, et al., 2008 with permission)

	Average foam volume per puncture, ml	Maximum foam volume per puncture, ml
Great saphenous vein	2-4	6
Small saphenous vein	2-4	4
Collateral veins	Up to 4	6
Recurrent varicose veins	Up to 4	8
Perforating veins	Up to 2	4
Reticular varicose veins	< 0.5	< 1
Spider veins	< 0.5	< 0.5
Venous malformations	2-6	< 8

Table 3. Preferred polidocanol concentration per injection
(From Breu FX, et al., 2008 with permission)

	Liquid	0.25%	0.5%	1%	2%	3%	4%
Great saphenous vein				+	++	++	
Small saphenous vein				+	++	+	
Collateral veins				++			
Recurrent varicose veins			(+)	++	++	+	
Perforating veins			(+)	++	+	(+)	
Reticular varicose veins	(+)	(+)	++	+			
Spider veins	++*	(+)*	(+)*				
Venous malformations			+	++	+		

Note: Concentrations given refer to liquid Polidocanol for conversion to a sclerosant foam.

++ indicates what most experts use to prepare foam for this indication.

+ indicates what is also used by experts, but less frequently than ++.

(+) indicates what is used by some or a few experts, or seldom.

++* For sclerotherapy of Tel with Polidocanol, it is recommended to use liquid sclerosant agents at first.

(+)* If foam is used, it is recommended to use small amounts of foam of 0.25%, or possibly 0.5%.

Body Position

Leg elevation during ultrasound-guided foam sclerotherapymay prevent foam from entering the deep venous system. When the leg is elevated, the foam will ascend to more distal parts of the vein, achieving eventualclosure of incompetent saphenous side branches or tributaries. At the FirstECMFS, a statement recommended elevation of the leg especially for treatment of larger veins.[20]Hill et al.[56]compared the utility of three commonly used techniques for reducing the migration of sclerosant foam during ultrasound-guided foam sclerotherapy: patient lying supine with application of digital pressure at the SFJ, elevation of the leg by 30 degrees with application of digital pressure at the SFJ, and elevation of the leg by 30 degrees without application of digital pressure at the SFJ.They concluded that ultrasound-guided foam sclerotherapy is best performed while the leg is elevated without digital pressure at the SFJ to avoid migration of the sclerosant foam. At the Second ECMFS, however, most participants considered that leg elevationduring foam sclerotherapy is notmandatory for safety reasons.[24]

Presence of Patent Foramen Ovale (PFO)

The known presence of a PFO indicates thatsclerotherapy must be performed with special caution. These patients should remain lyingdown for longer (8 to 30 minutes), only smallvolumesof foam (2 mL) orliquid sclerotherapy should be used, and the Valsalva maneuver should be avoided. [24]At the On-Line International Event on Sclerosing Foam and Patent Foramen Ovale, further procedures were recommended to prevent possible neurologic complications. These included requesting patients not to dress or put on their shoes and stockings by themselves, and ensuring that the patients were not constipatedbefore the procedure. However, the Committee did not reach a final conclusion as to whether there was a clear relationship between clinical events and the use of foam. While chronic cerebral damage resulting from PFO has been suggested, there has been no clear evidence of any acute cerebral effects resulting from injection of foam [57].

CONCLUSION

Since the introduction of sclerosing solution in foam sclerotherapy has rapidly gained popularity. Foam sclerotherapy is a safeand effective treatment for superficial truncalsaphenous incompetence as well as for varicose tributary veins. However, further studies may be necessary in order to devise better foam sclerotherapy techniques, including factors such as foam production, the optimal volume of foam, the use of physiologic gases, and more effective and safe injection techniques.

REFERENCES

[1] Kwaan JHK, Jones RN, Connolly JE. Simplified technique for the management of refractory varicose ulcers. *Surgery* 1976; 80: 743-747.

[2] D'Addato M. Gangrene of a limb with complete thrombosis of the venous system. *J. Cardiovasc. Surg.*(Torino) 1966; 7: 434-40.

[3] Sigg K. The treatment of varicosities and accompanying complications. *Angiolog.* 1952; 3: 355-79.

[4] Orbach EJ. A new approach to the sclerotherapy of varicose veins. *Angiology* 1950: 1; 302-5.

[5] Fegan WG. Continuous compression technique of injecting varicose veins. *Lancet* 1963: 20;2(7299): 109-12.

[6] McAusland S. The modern treatment of varicose veins. *Med. Press Circular.* 1939; 201: 404-10.

[7] Orbach EJ. Sclerotherapy of varicose veins – utilization of an intravenous air block. *Am. J. Surg.* 1944; LXVI (3): 362-6.

[8] Sigg K. Neuere gesichtspunkte zur Technik der Varizenbehandlung. *Ther. Umsch.* 1949; 6: 127-34.

[9] Orbach EJ. Contribution to the therapy of the varicose complex. *J. Int. Coll. Surg.* 1950; 13: 765-71.

[10] Cabrera J, Cabrera García-Olmedo J, Jr. Nuevo método de esclerosis en las varices tronculares. *Patologia Vascular.* 1995; 4: 55-73.

[11] Cabrera J, Cabrera J, Jr., Cabrera García-Olmedo MA. Élargissement des limites de la sclérothérapie: nouveaux produits sclérosants. *Phlébologie* 1997; 2: 181-8.

[12] Monfreux A. Traitement sclérosant des troncs saphéniens et leurs

collatérals de gros calible par la méthode MUS. *Phlébologie* 1997; 50: 351-3.

[13] Henriet JP. Un an de pratique quotidienne de la sclérothérapie par mousse de polidocanol (veines réticulares et télaniectasies): faisabilité, résultants, complications. *Phlébologie* 1997; 50: 355-60.

[14] Benigni JP, Sadoun S, Thirion V, Sica M, Demagny A, Chahim M. Foam of Lauromacrogol at 0.25% and treatment of telngiectasia and reticular veins. XIII World Congress of Phlebology, Sydney, 6-11 September 1998, 157.

[15] Benigni JP, Sadoun S, Thirion V, Sica M, Demagny A, Chahim M. Télangiectasies et varices réticulaires. Traitement par la mousse d'Aethoxysclérol à 0.25%. Présentation d'une étude pilote. *Phlébologie* 1999; 52: 283-9

[16] Mingo-Garcia J. Esclerosis venosa con espuma: Foam Medical System. *Revista Espanola de Medicina y Cirurgia Cosmetica.* 1997; 7: 29-31.

[17] Tessari L. Nouvelle technique d'obtention de la scléro-mousee. *Phlébologie* 2000; 53: 129.

[18] Sica M, Benigni JP. Échosclérose à la mousse: trios années d'expérience sur les axes saphéniens. *Phlébologie* 2000; 53: 339-42.

[19] Frullini A, Cavezzi A. Échosclérose par mousee de tétradécyl-sulfate de sodium et de polidocanol: deux années d'experience. *Phlébologie* 2000; 53: 431-5.

[20] Breu FX, Guggenbichler S. European consensus meeting on foam sclerotherapy, April 4-6, 2003, Tegernsee, Germany. *Dermatol. Surg.* 2004; 30: 709-17.

[21] Wollmann JC. The history of sclerosing foams. *Dermatol. Surg.*; 2004; 30: 694-703.

[22] Wollmann JC. Shaum-zwischen Vergangenheit und Zukunft. *Vasomed* 2002; 16: 34-5.

[23] Wollmann JC. Herstellung und Eigenschaften von Sklerosierungs schaum. *Vasomed* 2004; 16: 24.

[24] Breu FX, Guggenbichler S, Wollmann JC. 2nd European Consensus Meeting on Foam Sclerotherapy 2006, Tegernsee, Germany. *Vasa 2008;* S/71: 3-29.

[25] Coleridge-Smith P. Foam and liquid sclerotherapy for varicose veins. *Phlebology* 2009; 24 suppl 1: 62-72.

[26] Rabe E, Pannier-Fischer F, Gerlach H, Breu FX, Guggenbichler S, Zabel M. Guidelines for Sclerotherapy of Varicose Veins (ICD 10: I83.0,

I83.1, I83.2, and I83.9). *Dermatol. Surg.* 2004; 30: 687-93.

[27] Yamaki T, Nozaki M, Fujiwara O, Yoshida E. Comparative evaluation of duplex-derived parameters in patients with chronic venous insufficiency: correlation with clinical manifestations. *J. Am. Coll. Surg.* 2002; 195: 822-30.

[28] Walsh JC, Bergan JJ, Beeman S, Comer TP. Femoral venous reflux abolished by greater saphenous vein stripping. *Ann. Vasc. Surg.* 1994 ; 8 : 566-70

[29] Sales CM, Bilof ML, Petrillo KA, Luka NL. Correction of lower extremity deep venous incompetence by ablation of superficial venous reflux. *Ann. Vasc. Surg.* 1996 ; 10 : 186-9.

[30] Yamaki T, Nozaki M, Sasaki K. Quantitative assessment of superficial venous insufficiency using duplex ultrasound and air plethysmography. *Dermatol. Surg.* 2000; 26: 644-648.

[31] Yamaki T, Nozaki M, Sakurai H, Takeuchi M, Kono T, Soejima K. Quantification of venous reflux parameters using duplex scanning and air plethysmograpy. *Phlebology* 2007; 22: 20-8.

[32] Schadeck M. Ultrasound guided sclerotherapy In: Schadeck M, ed. Duplex and Phlebology. Napoli: *Gnocchi*, 1994: 115-28.

[33] Zummo M, Forrestal M. Sclerotherapy of the long saphenous vein: a prospective duplex controlled comparative study. *Phlebology* 1994; Suppl. 1: 571-3.

[34] Bishop CCR, Fronek HS, Fronek A, Dilley RB, Bernstein. Real-time color duplex scanning after sclerotherapy of the greater saphenous vein. *J. Vasc. Surg.* 1991; 14: 505-10.

[35] Kanter A, Thibault P. Saphenofemoral incompetence treated by ultrasound-guided sclerotherapy. *Dermatol. Surg.* 1996; 22: 648-52.

[36] Baccaglini U, Spreafico G, Castoro C, Sorrentino P. Consensus conference on varicose veins of lower extremity. *Phlebology* 1997; 12: 2-16

[37] Hamel-Desnos C, Desnos P, Wollman JC, Ouvry P, Mako S, Allaert FA. Evaluation of the efficacy of polidocanol in the form of foam compared with liquid form in sclerotherapy of the greater saphenous vein: initial results. *Dermatol. Surg.* 2003; 29: 1170-5.

[38] Yamaki T, Nozaki M, Iwasaka S. Comparative study of duplex-guided foam sclerotherapy and duplex-guided liquid sclerotherapy for the treatment of superficial venous insufficiency. *Dermatol. Surg.* 2004; 30: 718-22.

[39] Rabe E, Otto J, Schliephake D, Pannier F. Efficacy and safety of great

saphenous vein sclerotherapy using standardised polidocanol foam (ESAF): a randomised controlled multicentre clinical trial. *Eur. J. Vasc. Endovasc. Surg.* 2008; 35: 238-45.

[40]   Ouvry P, Allaert FA, Desnos P, Hamel-Desnos C. Efficacyof polidocanol foam versus liquid in sclerotherapy of thegreat saphenous vein: a multicentre randomised controlledtrial with a 2-year follow-up. *Eur. J. Vasc. Endovasc.Surg.* 2008;36:366-70.

[41]   Myers KA, Jolley D, Clough A, Kirwan J. Outcome of ultrasound-guided sclerotherapy for varicose veins: medium-term results assessed by ultrasound surveillance. *Eur. J. Vasc. Endovasc. Surg.* 2007; 33: 116-21.

[42]   Wright D, Gobin JP, Bradbury AW, Coleridge-Smith P, Spoelstra H, Berridge D, Wittens CHA, Sommer A, Nelzen O, Chanter D. Varisolve® European Phase III Investigators Group. Varisolve polidocanol microfoam compared with surgery or sclerotherapy in the management of varicose veins in the presence of trunk vein incompetence: European randomized controlled trial. *Phlebology* 2006; 21: 180-90.

[43]   Bountouroglou DG, Azzam M, Kakkos SK Pathmarajah M, Young P, Geroulakos G. Ultrasound-guided foam sclerotherapy combined with sapheno-femoral ligation compared to surgical treatment of varicose veins: early resultsof arandomized controlledtrial.*Eur.J. Vasc. Endovasc. Surg.*2006; 31: 93-100.

[44]   Gonzalez-Zeh R, Armisen R, Barahona S. Endovenouslaser and echo-guided foam ablation in great saphenousvein reflux: one-year follow-up results. *J. Vasc. Surg.*2008; 48: 940-6.

[45]   van den Bos R, Arends L, Kockaert M, Neumann M, Nijsten T. Endovenous therapies of lower extremity varicosities: a meta-analysis. *J. Vasc. Surg.* 2009; 49: 230-9.

[46]   Guex JJ, Allaert FA, Gillet JL, Chleir F. Immediate and midterm complications of sclerotherapy: report of a prospective multicenter registry of 12,173 sclerotherapy sessions. *Dermatol. Surg.* 2005; 31: 123-8.

[47]   Alòs J, Carreño P, López JA, Estadella B, Serra-Prat M, Marinel-lo J. Efficacy and safety of sclerotherapy using polidocanol foam: a controlled clinical trial. *Eur. J. Vasc. Endovasc. Surg.* 2006; 31: 101-7.

[48]   Hanisch F, Muller T, Krivokuca M, Winterholler M. Stroke following variceal sclerotherapy. *Eur. J. Med. Res.* 2004; 9: 282-4.

[49] Forlee MV, Grouden M, Moore DJ, Shanik G. Stroke after varicose vein foam injection sclerotherapy. *J. Vasc. Surg.* 2006; 43: 162-4.

[50] Eckmann DM, Kobayashi S, Li M. Microvascular embolization following microfoam sclerosant administration. *Dermatol. Surg.* 2005; 31: 636-43.

[51] Morrison N, Neuhardt DL, Rogers CR, McEown J, Morrison T, Johnson E, Salles-Cunha SX. Comparisons of side effects using air and carbon dioxide foam for endovenous chemical ablation. *J. Vasc. Surg.* 2008; 47: 830-6.

[52] Bhowmick A, Harper D, Wright D, McCollum CN. Polidocanol microfoam sclerotherapy for longsaphenous varicose veins.*Phlebology* 2001; 16: 41-50.

[53] McCollum C, Bhowmick A, Harper D. UK experience withVarisolve Polidocanol microfoam. *Int. Angiol.* 2001; 20(Suppl 1): 86.

[54] Myers KA, Jolley D, Clough A, Kirwan J. Outcome of ultrasound-guided sclerotherapy for varicose veins: medium-term results assessed by ultrasound surveillance. *Eur. J. Vasc. Endovasc. Surg.* 2007; 33: 116-21.

[55] Yamaki T,Nozaki M, Sakurai H, Takeuchi M, Soejima K, Kono T. Multiple small-dose injections can reduce the passage of sclerosant foam into deep veins during foam sclerotherapy for varicose veins. *Eur. J. Vasc. Endovasc. Surg.*2009; 37: 343-8.

[56] Hill D, Hamilton R, Fung T. Assessment of techniques to reduce sclerosant foam migration during ultrasound-guided sclerotherapy of the great saphenous vein. *J. Vasc. Surg.* 2008; 48: 934-9.

[57] Passariello F. Sclerosing foam and patent foramen ovale. The final report. *Intern. Angiol.* 2007; 26 (Suppl 1): 87.

In: Varicose Veins
Editor: Andrea L. Nelson

ISBN 978-1-61209-841-8
©2011 Nova Science Publishers, Inc.

Chapter 5

AIRPLETHYSMOGRAPHY: A DIAGNOSTIC TECHNIQUE

Ui-Jun Park[1] and Dong-Ik Kim[2]

[1]Keimyung University and [2]Sungkyunkwan University School of Medicine, Korea

INTRODUCTION

The objectives of the examination of venous abnormalities are to determine whether the problem is the result of outflow obstruction, reflux, or both, and to define the anatomic location; in addition, quantitative hemodynamic information is generally collected. Duplex ultrasonography is a useful test for the evaluation of reflux and obstruction of individual veins; however, it provides little quantitative hemodynamic information.

The ambulatory venous pressure (AVP) is the gold standard for functional and quantitative testing of the venous system of the lower extremities. The AVP is obtained by placing a catheter into a superficial vein of the lower leg. Pressure changes are recorded while the patient exercises the calf muscle pump by walking, rising up on tiptoes, or performing ankle dorsiflexion movement. Direct measurement of the AVP is the most reliable way to evaluate venous function; however, it is rarely used in clinical practice because of its invasive and time-consuming requirements. Instead, various plethysmography (air, strain gauge, impedance, photo) techniques have been developed for clinical use with the aim of replacing AVP measurements; plethysmograpic techniques quantitate the degree of reflux, obstruction, and/or calf muscle dysfunction by measuring changes in calf volume on various maneuvers.

Strain plethysmography measures the electrical resistance and is plotted on a strip chart, using a mercury strain gauge placed around the extremity. Change in volume causes a change in circumference and therefore in the length and electrical resistance of the strain. Impedance plethysmography measures the electrical impedance, which is inversely proportional to the volume. Photo plethysmography measures the reflection of infrared light by red blood cells in the cutaneous capillaries. Dorsal or plantar flexion of the foot reduces the amount of blood in the dermal plexus. On cessation of exercise, photoplethysmography records the capillary refilling time related to the dermal circulation. Airplethysmography (APG) is a technique used for measuring the pressure or volume changes in the lower limb using an air chamber placed around the lower leg.

AIRPLETHSMOGRAPHY

In the 1960s, Allan described changes in the leg vein volume that occur as a result of the development of varicose disease.[1] This prior work has led to the development of the modern airplethysmograph, which is available for use clinically. The APG was first introduced by Christopoulos et al. as a tool for assessing global venous function of the lower extremity. The APG measures various parameters such as venous volume, the venous filling index, the ejection fraction and the residual volume fraction. The results of the APG correlate well with the AVP and it is useful for diagnosis and quantification of venous reflux and for the evaluation of the clinical severity of chronic venous insufficiency.[2,3] It provides reproducible hemodynamic measurements that can be evaluated noninvasively in serial examinations.

EQUIPMENT AND EXAMINATION TECHNIQUE

The APG consists of an air chamber (leg sensing cuff) that surrounds the whole leg, a calibration syringe, a main control unit, and a computer system. The patient is placed in the supine position with the knee of the examined leg slightly flexed and the heel on a support: The air chamber is placed on the calf, which wraps around the whole length of the calf, and then the zipper is closed and is placed on the anterior side of the leg. (Figure 1)

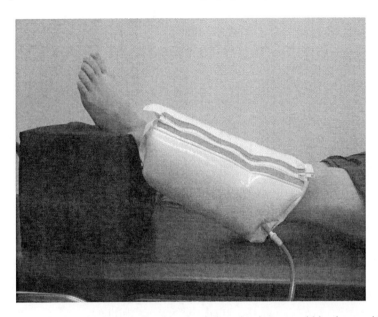

Figure 1. The air chamber is an inflatable plastic bag that is trapezoid in shape with the upper part wider than the lower part, and can be fixed with a zipper. It is also suitable for wrapping the whole length of the calf and is 14 inches or 10 inches in size.

Next, the system should be calibrated. The air chamber is inflated with air to 6mmHg and connected to the main control unit and computer system. A calibration syringe (100mL) is placed between the air chamber and the main control unit with a T shaped tube and is used for calibration. Calibration is performed by depressing the plunger of the syringe, compressing the air included in the airplethysmograph, reducing its volume by 100mL, and evaluating the corresponding pressure change. After calibration the plunger is pulled back to its original position when the pressure in the air chamber returns to 6 mmHg. The pressure of 6 mmHg has been selected because it is the lowest pressure that ensures good contact between the air chamber and the limb with minimum compression of the veins. If the air chamber inflating pressure was too low, it could not conduct the venous calf pressure exactly; whereas, if the air chamber inflating pressure is too high, it would compress the superficial venous system. Tissue movement during changes in posture and exercise are unlikely to interfere with the measurement because the air chamber includes almost all of the tissues from the knee to the ankle.

The patient is fitted with the air chamber and the leg is elevated to about 45 degrees.(Figure 2-A, 3-A) After emptying the venous blood from the leg, and a stable baseline is reached, the patient steps down from the examination table carefully without putting any weight on the leg being studied. Then the parameters are recorded. Because every external pressure that touches the air chamber is recognized as information that increases the venous pressure, movements that touch the air chamber must be prohibited until the examination is completed. The patient is directed to stand on the support safely so as not to fall.

The venous volume (VV), the venous filling time and the venous filling index (VFI) on standing when getting up from the recumbent position are measured. The rising curve on the monitor is proportional to the increase in calf venous pressure; the patient is kept in the same position until the rising curve reaches a stable plateau. This point indicates the maximal venous volume of the calf vein. If the rising curve reaches the maximal volume sooner than the optimal time, this means that there is venous regurgitation from venous valvular insufficiency. The time in seconds required to reach a stable plateau on the APG test is called the venous filling time, and the VFI is calculated by dividing the VV at 90% refilling by the venous filling time required to reach 90% refilling.(Figure 2-B, 3-B).

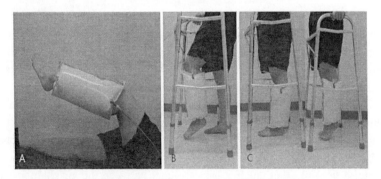

Figure 2. A. the leg is elevated to about 45 degrees, with the knee of the examined leg kept slightly flexed and not touching the air chamber; B. The patient stands on the floor holding the support without putting any weight on the leg being studied. C. The patient puts the same weight on both legs and raises the heel slowly as high as possible, and then flexes the knee and goes back to the first position with the leg flexed and the foot raised. During this examination, the air chamber should not be compressed by the contralateral leg, any support or the examination table.

After this, the EF and RVF are examined. The patient raises the heel slowly as high as possible, and then flexes the knee and goes back to the first position with the leg flexed and the foot raised.(Figure 2-C) This causes the calf muscles to contract, and the intramuscular venous flow to eject to the thigh. The graph on the monitor falls in proportion to the ejected venous flow caused by raising the calf. If the leg goes back to the initial position, the graph rises to the highest point. The ejected volume (EV) was measured and the ejection fraction (EF = EV×100/VV) was calculated with one tiptoe movement. (Figure 3-C)

In a similar manner, the residual volume and residual volume fraction (RVF = RV×100/VV) after 10 tiptoe movements, are measured. The patient raises the heel as soon as possible. This exercise is repeated ten times. The point that indicates the greatest fall on the graph represents the residual calf volume.(Figure 3-D).

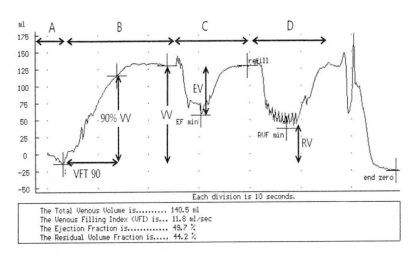

Figure 3. APG recording of volume changes during the sequence of postural changes and exercise in a patient with varicose veins: A. emptying the venous blood from the leg; B. venous filling; C. one tiptoe movement; D. ten consecutive tiptoe movements: VV, venous volume; VFT, venous filling time; EV, ejection volume; RV, residual volume; VFI=90% VV/VFT 90; Ejection Fraction (EF)=EV100/VV; Residual volume fraction (RVF) = RV100/VV: A. emptying the venous blood from the leg; B. venous filling; C. one tiptoe movement; D. ten consecutive tiptoe movements.

INTERPRETATION OF APG RESULTS

APG allows the detection of volume changes of the lower extremity induced by gravity or exercise. APG quantifies the physiologic components of chronic venous insufficiency: chronic obstruction, valvular insufficiency, calf muscle pump function, and venous hypertension. APG can measure the actual blood volume changes in milliliters and blood flow in milliliters per second. Measurements of venous hemodynamics are obtained directly or calculated from the volume data.

The VV is for the amount of blood in the venous reservoir of the lower leg. It is increased in the leg with obstruction or reflux and it can be reduced with optimal treatment.[4-6] The functional VV ranges from 100-150mL in normal limbs and reaches up to 350mL in limbs with venous disease.[7] Because of the variation in leg size, the volume measurements (VV, EV, and RV) expressed in absolute units (milliliters) vary with each individual and largely depend on the body mass; these measures are less useful clinically except for the longitudinal surveillance of treatment in a given patient. The VFI, EF and RVF, indexed to the venous volume as a ratio, are useful parameters as objective assessments independent of variations in the size of the leg. The VFI measures the venous refilling rate of the calf, thereby assessing the overall degree of venous reflux. The VFI is less than 2mL/sec in normal limbs and increases up to 30mL/sec in limbs with venous reflux. The measurement of VFI can be repeated after resolution of reflux in the superficial veins at the level of the knee, using tourniquets. The VFI is reduced to less than 5mL/sec in limbs with primary varicose veins and competent deep venous valves, however, not in limbs with reflux in the deep venous system.[8] After treatment of insufficiency of the superficial venous system, venous reflux measured as the VFI is also reduced.[4] The VFI is a parameter highly correlated with the clinical severity of venous disease.[5,7,9]

The EV is the amount of blood ejected as a result of a single calf muscle contraction. The EV is about 100mL in normal limbs but less in limbs with deep venous disease; this is because of obstruction of deep vein or retrograde ejection via incompetent perforating veins. Normal limbs have an EF greater than 60%, and an EF less than 40% is considered abnormal.[7] The residual volume fraction affects venous reflux, obstruction and ejection capacity of the calf muscle pump; it is calculated from the residual volume after 10 tiptoe movements. In normal limbs the RVF is less than 35%; however, it is increased in limbs with impaired venous emptying. After the first few tiptoe movements, a steady state is achieved, because the amount of blood expelled from the veins of the leg, as a result of each calf muscle contraction, is the same as the amount of blood entering during each period of relaxation from venous reflux. The EF and RVF assess the function of the calf muscle pump and they are related to the incidence of ulceration.[9-12] The RVF is highly correlated with ambulatory venous pressures.[9]

CLINICAL APPLICATION OF THE APG

In chronic venous insufficiency, the APG can be used to help determine the appropriate patient management. Unique to the APG is its ability to quantify whole limb reflux in mLs per second as well as the calf muscle pump function. Both the amount of reflux and the efficiency of the calf muscle pump function are related to venous disease. Several studies have attempted to determine the role of the APG in the diagnosis of chronic venous insufficiency.[13-15] The APG has been found to be a reasonable method for determining the presence or absence of chronic venous insufficiency. An increase in the VFI of more than 2mL/s is associated with chronic venous insufficiency.

Although there have been attempts to investigate the value of the APG with regard to its correlation with the clinical severity of disease and the anatomic distribution of reflux, the results of studies have been inconsistent. Some investigators failed to show differences in the APG parameters for various categories of chronic venous insufficiency[13,15,16]; however, others report that the VFI is a good predictor of venous reflux, is a good determinant of the clinical severity of venous disease, and offers some degree of prediction for perforator and deep vein reflux.[9]

Objective, long term follow up can be provided because of the noninvasive, repeatable, operator independent measurements of the APG. APG testing has been used not only to diagnose venous disease but also to obtain an objective measure of the changes in venous hemodynamics after therapeutic interventions in patients with chronic venous insufficiency. One of the advantages of the APG is that it can be used over an elastic stocking. One study demonstrated that improvement of APG parameters was documented in lower extremities with chronic venous insufficiency treated with compression stockings.[2] Functional VV is reduced and venous reflux, indicated by changes of the VFI, is also reduced by elastic compression. The most pronounced effect of elastic stockings is shown by changes in the RVF. These findings indicate that the APG is a practical noninvasive method that can assess the effect of elastic compression.

The APG can be used to assess the results and prognosis of surgical intervention in a patient.[2,4,6,17] In one study, analysis of the postoperative hemodynamic changes in 1,756 limbs, undergoing varicose vein surgery using the APG, showed that the hemodynamic parameters were significantly improved after surgery in terms of a decrease in the VV, VFI, RVF and an increase in the EF.[18] (Figure 4).

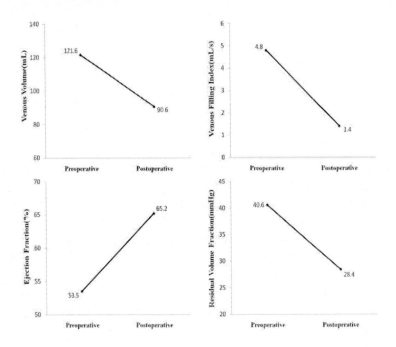

Figure 4. Changes of the hemodynamic parameters before and after surgery of primary varicose veins: Preoperatively, the median VV 121.6 (94.7- 160.6) mL, the median VFI 4.8 (2.9-7.6) mL/s, the median RVF 40.6 (29.7-50.0)% and the median EF 53.5 (44.3-64.1)%. Postoperatively, the median VV 90.6 (69.1-116.8) mL, the median VFI 1.4 (0.9-1.9) mL/s, the median RVF 28.4 (17.5-38.7)% and the median EF 65.2 (54.5-77.2)%. The VV, VFI and RVF were reduced 25.2%, 71.5% and 29.9%, respectively. The EF was increased 20.3%. The results were significant for all four variables (P <.001).

The overall hemodynamic changes were plotted on the graph in relation to the EF and VFI. Although all of the limbs were not normalized after surgery, the majority of the limbs shifted in a hemodynamically favorable direction after surgery. With these results, venous reflux and calf muscle pump function were grossly improved after surgery.(Figure 5)

APG is easily performed and tolerated by patients. It provides valuable information on the impact of reflux and obstruction on overall venous function, and can provide a measure of the calf muscle pump function. The APG can be used as a screening test for venous disease, and it is useful for the assessment of objective hemodynamic improvement after treatment of venous disease. The use of APG as a complementary modality to duplex ultrasound is reasonable for quantification of reflux or obstruction, for monitoring of dynamics of venous disease over time and for evaluation of treatment outcomes.

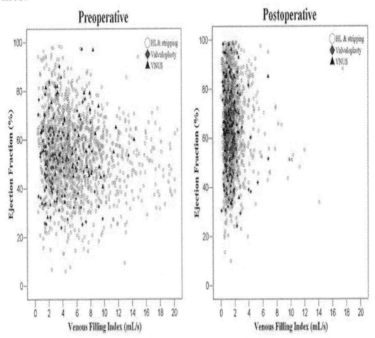

Figure 5. A scatter plot showing hemodynamic changes in the EF and VFI: The majority of dots are in the right lower quadrant preoperatively. These dots are shifted to the left upper quadrant. Among all limbs, the percent of cases with a VFI of more than 2mL/s was 89% preoperatively; it was improved after surgery so that the percent of cases with a VFI less than 2mL/s was 74%: HL and stripping, high ligation and stripping of the GSV with varicosectomy; Valvuloplasty, Valvuloplasty of the GSV with varicosectomy; VNUS, obliteration of the GSV using VNUS system and varicosectomy.

REFERENCES

[1]   Allan J. volume changes in the lower limb in response to postural alterations and muscular exercise. *S Afr j Surg* 1963;2:75-90.

[2]   Christopoulos DG, Nicolaides AN, Szendro G, Irvine AT, Bull ML, Eastcott HH. Air-plethysmography and the effect of elastic compression on venous hemodynamics of the leg. *J Vasc Surg* 1987;5:148-59.

[3]   Nicolaides AN. Investigation of Chronic *Venous Insufficiency : A Consensus Statement. Circulation* 2000;102:e126-63.

[4]   Christopoulos D, Nicolaides AN, Galloway JM, Wilkinson A. Objective noninvasive evaluation of venous surgical results. *J Vasc Surg* 1988;8:683-7.

[5]   Owens LV, Farber MA, Young ML, Carlin RE, Criado-Pallares E, Passman MA, et al. The value of air plethysmography in predicting clinical outcome after surgical treatment of chronic venous insufficiency. *J Vasc Surg* 2000;32:961-8.

[6]   Gillespie DL, Cordts PR, Hartono C, Woodson J, Obi-Tabot E, LaMorte WW, et al. The role of air plethysmography in monitoring results of venous surgery. *J Vasc Surg* 1992;16:674-8.

[7]   Christopoulos D, Nicolaides AN, Szendro G. Venous reflux: quantification and correlation with the clinical severity of chronic venous disease. *Br J Surg* 1988;75:352-6.

[8]   Christopoulos D, Nicolaides AN. Noninvasive diagnosis and quantitation of popliteal reflux in the swollen and ulcerated leg. *J Cardiovasc Surg (Torino)* 1988;29:535-9.

[9]   Criado E, Farber MA, Marston WA, Daniel PF, Burnham CB, Keagy BA. The role of air plethysmography in the diagnosis of chronic venous insufficiency. *Journal of Vascular Surgery* 1998;27:660-70.

[10] Padberg JFT, Pappas PJ, Araki CT, Back TL, Hobson Ii RW. Hemodynamic and clinical improvement after superficial vein ablation in primary combined venous insufficiency with ulceration. *Journal of Vascular Surgery* 1996;24:711-8.

[11] Miyazaki K, Nishibe T, Kudo F, Miyazaki YJ, Nishibe M, Ando M, et al. Hemodynamic changes in stripping operation or saphenofemoral ligation of the greater saphenous vein for primary varicose veins. *Ann Vasc Surg* 2004;18:465-9.

[12] Yamaki T, Nozaki M, Sakurai H, Takeuchi M, Kono T, Soejima K.
      Quantification of venous reflux parameters using duplex scanning and
      air plethysmography. *Phlebology* 2007;22:20-8.
[13] Nishibe T, Kudo F, Miyazaki K, Kondo Y, Nishibe M, Dardik A.
      Relationship between air-plethysmographic venous function and clinical
      severity in primary varicose veins. *Int Angiol* 2006;25:352-5.
[14] Nishibe T, Kudo F, Miyazaki K, Kondo Y, Nishibe M, Muto A, et al.
      Relationship between parameters of air plethysmography and types of
      superficial venous reflux in patients with primary varicose veins. *Int
      Angiol* 2008;27:385-8.
[15] Iafrati MD, Welch H, O'Donnell TF, Belkin M, Umphrey S,
      McLaughlin R. Correlation of venous noninvasive tests with the Society
      for Vascular Surgery/International Society for Cardiovascular Surgery
      clinical classification of chronic venous insufficiency. *J Vasc Surg*
      1994;19:1001-7.
[16] van Bemmelen PS, Mattos MA, Hodgson KJ, Barkmeier LD, Ramsey
      DE, Faught WE, et al. Does air plethysmography correlate with duplex
      scanning in patients with chronic venous insufficiency? *J Vasc Surg*
      1993;18:796-807.
[17] Welkie JF, Comerota AJ, Kerr RP, Katz ML, Jayheimer EC, Brigham
      RA. The hemodynamics of venous ulceration. *Ann Vasc Surg* 1992;6:1-
      4.
[18] Park UJ, Yun WS, Lee KB, Rho YN, Kim YW, Joh JH, et al. Analysis
      of the postoperative hemodynamic changes in varicose vein surgery
      using air plethysmography. *J Vasc Surg*;51:634-8.

In: Varicose Veins   ISBN 978-1-61209-841-8
Editor: Andrea L. Nelson   ©2011 Nova Science Publishers, Inc.

Chapter 6

THE CHALLENGE OF UPWARD VS DOWNWARD DEVELOPMENT OF PRIMARY VARICOSE VEINS

Paola De Rango[1] and Paolo Bonanno

Vascular and Endovascular Division, Hospital S.M. Misericordia,
Perugia, Italy

ABSTRACT

Despite primary venous insufficiency is one of the most common diseases, pathophysiology leading to varicose vein development is today not well understood and object of multiple conjectures. Unfortunately, due to the complexity in investigating a dynamic phenomenon with multiple evolutions, dissimilar populations and incomparable settings, large longitudinal studies on the natural history of varicose veins are lacking and the mechanisms behind the development and progression of reflux in primary superficial venous insufficiency still remain largely uncertain.

Over the years, diverging theoretical models based on multiple assumptions have been developed to explain the relationship between venous reflux and venous disease, one of the most debated issues being whether development of varicose veins occurs downward or upraises along the leg. This understanding has indeed relevant implications for

---

[1] Corresponding Author: Paola De Rango, MD, Vascular and Endovascular Division, Hospital S.M. Misericordia, University of Perugia, 06129, Perugia, Italy. Phone: +39 075-5786440. Fax: +39 075-5786435. Email: plderango@gmail.com , pderango@unipg.it.

treatment, since the initial ("starting") points of venous disease are usually the most severe compromised necessitating of more aggressive and earlier treatment. At the opposite, the last involved venous sites might not require any direct action since the disease can spontaneously reverse once the treatment is applied to the first and more severe involved points. Therefore, dissimilar theoretical models on varicose vein progression have provided opposite basis for the development of new and improvement of existing therapies. Today large open debate in the varicose vein pathophysiology field, where traditional and modern concepts oppose, still remains. Critical analysis of evidence is essential to support scientific progress and objectively understand which and on what extent each theory might be reliable.

The long-standing traditional concepts, suggesting varicose vein as a primary disease at the terminal valve that develops downwards along the limbs ("retrograde theory"), are still the most believed hypotheses. This traditional theory was mainly empirical and based on animal models and grossly pathology observations. Since it was known from Harvey's experiments that in normal veins blood flows in unidirectional way, when Brodie and Trendelemburg' observations showed that this unidirectionality was disrupted in extremities with varicose veins, it was logical to infer causality.[1] However, causality of valve incompetence that leads the development of reflux remains still far to be demonstrated and so too the mechanisms involved in the relationship between venous reflux and venous disease.

Indeed, more recent advances in imaging (especially ultrasound) and better understanding in histology, biochemical and genetic markers have progressively and increasingly raised skepticism about the original Trendelemburg-based theory. More than one reason to support an opposite pathophysiology with a reverse, upward development of the venous disease has been moved.

The innovative explanation of venous reflux as an ascending phenomenon starting from the distal leg and uprising up to the terminal valve ("ascending theory") was increasingly reinforced by a number of convincing research findings. At the opposite, the old-standing interpretation of venous reflux as a retrograde downward phenomenon appears still today weakly reasonable and not sustained by strong basic research and clinical data.

The first findings against the traditional theory arose from many biochemical and histology researches on vessel wall and endothelium suggesting that changes in the vein wall with "wall weakening" more than primary valve damage could be the first stage of a disease predisposing to vein dilation and incompetence.

Furthermore, it was also noted that the traditional believed causality of valve incompetence hypothesis contrasted with basic physic laws and gravity forces. It was difficult to reasonably explain why should venous disease firstly occur where venous stasis is less relevant because of lower gravitational force, and lower hydrostatic pressure and, therefore, why the incompetence of junctional sapheno-femoral valves should be the initiating factor in promoting reflux in a primary venous disease that develops in a retrograde anti-gravitational fashion along limb veins. Since the venous stasis is obviously higher at the bottom of the hydrostatic pressure column of blood where the gravity force is stronger, it is more likely that, as a manifestation of venous stasis, venous incompetence will be firstly recorded at distal points of the limb where the pressure is higher. From these points, with the progressing of the disease and the advancing of venous stasis, hyper-pressure might subsequently rise following the gravity gradient (higher at the bottom, lighter at the top of the hydrostatic pressure column) promoting dilatation and incompetence of vein leaflets to upper levels. The last to be involved would be the junction.

Therefore, biochemical, hemodynamic and physical principles all can support that the natural history of venous insufficiency follows an "ascending evolution", that is, the disease likely begins at the lower levels of the limbs and develops in an antegrade manner. The causality of valve incompetence supporting a retrograde theory of reflux evolution remains, with respect to physic laws, largely speculative and lacks of biochemical strong substrate.

Finally, the "causality" of valve incompetence does also difficulty match the well-known findings of reflux of great saphenous vein occurring with total competence at the saphenous- femoro confluence (as described in about 50% of varicose saphenous veins). It is indeed a common finding in clinical practice that varicosities on lower limbs are most often seen in the medial and postero-medial aspect of the calf. Ultrasound mapping studies have shown that the most common patterns of varicose veins are in the calf. Because of the increased hydrostatic pressure levels, the lowest limb level represents not only the starting point but also the point of more severe reflux responsible for developing the earliest symptoms and signs of venous insufficiency. The continuous increase in hydrostatic pressure allows progressive enlargement and valve insufficiency of the above venous axis that, if not treated, will propagate upwards following the hydrostatic pressure gradient, and finally will involve the terminal valve at junctions in a later time. Again, the terminal saphenous-femoral confluence valve is most likely the last and not the first to be involved from a disease that ascends.

According to these 3 news observations (wall weakening, physic laws and venous incompetence with saphenous- femoral valve competence preservation) the following model of venous pathophysiology ("ascending theory") was therefore inferred. Incompetent valve results from changes and dilatation in the vein wall; wall weakening is the predisposing factor, necessary but not sufficient by itself to decompensate the venous system that requires the overlapping of venous hyper-pressure. Venous pressure applies along the venous axis following the gravitational gradient, therefore allowing higher venous stasis at the bottom (distal leg) where venous system earlier decompensates, dilates and becomes incompetent. According to the distribution of venous pressure, wall vein weakening will subsequently decompensate, progressively, along the pressure column. Only huge and sustained pressure can develop incompetence at the junctional valve in subsequent and more advanced times. Incompetent junctions are indeed often described in older patients with longer-standing disease and multifocal disease as an expression of later stages of venous insufficiency more than an initial step. [2-4]

Accepting the retrograde hypothesis one cannot believe to the benefit of preservation of a refluxing saphenous junction during treatment of varicose veins as it has been indeed recently demonstrated by a number of studies analyzing approaches for management of varicose veins without intervention on the junction. If the valve is the starting point of the disease, any treatment, to be effective, should be performed at this level: without this first step the disease could not be cured. At the opposite, a number of different sparing-valve techniques, either extensive ablative or super-selective and more conservative, have been recently successfully applied for treatment of venous insufficiencies. The common finding of studies supporting these techniques was the possibility of junctional valve incompetence recovery in most cases as hemodynamic consequence of procedures performed in venous segments located below the junction and without any direct action on the junctional valve. The treatment (sclerotherapy or ligation) has been directed on the sub-junctional saphenous vein (either collaterals or saphenous trunk) or has been entirely performed outside the saphenous axis allowing, in any cases, an effective venous drainage. This clearly demonstrated that the valve was not the promoting essential factor in varicose veins but a consequence of a pathology process starting at different levels and involving the junction only with time at delayed stages.

It is remarkable that two new specific venous techniques, based on completely different and even conflicting approaches to venous diseases, both provided evidence in favor of the ascending theory in the recent years.[5-8] Pittaluga et al, offered the technique of extensive ablation of venous reservoir (extensive phlebectomies and stripping) without actions on the saphenous-femoral confluence, the Ambulatory Selective Varices Ablation under Local Anesthesia (ASVAL), as an effective tool to reverse at 4 years symptoms and reflux in 65% of limbs with saphenous refluxing junctions.[5-6] The basic concepts of ASVAL were to exclude all reflux points by extensive ablation of all superficial varicosities (mainly tributary veins) while preserving the saphenous–femoral confluence to allow drainage from groin collaterals into the deep circulation. [9]

The second innovative sparing-valve venous technique was more conservative and used sclerotherapy.[7-8] Superselective application of sclerotherapy below the junctional valve into a saphenous segment (Echo-Sclerosis haEmodynamic Conservative: ESEC 1 technique) or into a saphenous branch (ESEC 2 technique or indirect technique) over a confluence point was successful applied in 90% of varicose limbs with benefit persisting in the long term (14 years). An interesting finding of ESEC study was that the terminal valve incompetence at the saphenous junction recovered when the sub-junctional saphenous vein shrank after the interruption of the hydrostatic weight pressure at a below level. The principles of ESEC were indeed based on the effects of the breakage of the hydrostatic pressure column by sclerosis to decrease the amount of venous pressure and to allow venous drainage at the confluence points and into the deep system through perforator veins (reentry points). Breakage of the single column indeed allows to obtain two columns, each at lower pressure. The decreased pressure along the hydrostatic column allows shrinkage of the previously dilated vein (because previously hyper-pressurized) with recovery of the valve function. Authors of ESEC found that sclerotherapy applied in the selected vein segment was followed by the shrinkage of the venous trunk above with recovered continence. Similarly, treatment applied in the saphenous trunk (or in a saphenous tributary) below the junctional level could allow the recovery of the junctional valve and the shrinkage of the saphenous junction.[7-8]

Although it is still challenging to demonstrate, there are today more and better-evidenced factors supporting an upward than a downward development of reflux in primary venous insufficiency of lower limbs.
This pathophysiology pattern should be taken into account in evaluating treatment plans for patients with venous insufficiency.

Today the management of varicose disease is not standardized and largely based on a variety of approaches and treatments also because of the lack of demonstrated superiority of each treatment strategy. Nevertheless, varicose veins are one of the most common progressive diseases with inevitable chronic evolution. Complete recovery from the disease, as well as the absolute prevention of recurrences, are clearly impossible. However, the best evidenced research and future studies are essential to find out and possibly uniform the best way to improve the consequence of this disorder that also implies relevant society health burden and costs.

REFERENCES

[1] Lurie F. Venous haemodynamics: what we know and don't know. *Phlebology.* 2009;24:3-7.
[2] Labropoulos N, Giannoukas AD, Delis K, Mansour MA, Kang SS, Nicolaides AN, Lumley J, Baker WH. Where does venous reflux start? *J. Vasc. Surg.* 1997 Nov;26(5):736-42.
[3] Caggiati A, Rosi C, Heyn R, Franceschini M, Acconcia MC. Age-related variations of varicose veins anatomy. *J. Vasc. Surg.* 2006 Dec; 44(6):1291-5.
[4] Wong JK, Duncan JL, Nichols DM. Whole-leg duplex mapping for varicose veins: observations on patterns of reflux in recurrent and primary legs, with clinical correlation. *Eur. J. Vasc. Endovasc. Surg.* 2003 Mar;25(3):267-75.
[5] Pittaluga P, Chastanet S, Guex JJ. Great saphenous vein stripping with preservation of sapheno-femoral confluence: hemodynamic and clinical results. *J. Vasc. Surg.* 2008 Jun;47(6):1300-4.
[6] Pittaluga P, Chastanet S, Rea B, Barbe R. Midterm results of the surgical treatment of varices by phlebectomy with conservation of a refluxing saphenous vein. *J. Vasc. Surg.* 2009 Jul;50(1):107-18.
[7] Bernardini E, Piccioli R, De Rango P, Bisacci C, Pagliuca V, Bisacci R. Ambulatory and hemodynamic treatment of venous insufficiency by ultrasound-guided sclerotherapy: 14 year results. *Phlebologie* 2007; 4:186-195.
[8] Bernardini E, Piccioli R, De Rango P, Bisacci C, Pagliuca V, Bisacci R. Echo-sclerosis hemodynamic conservative: a new technique for varicose vein treatment. *Ann. Vasc. Surg.* 2007 Jul;21(4):535-43.

[9]   Muller R. Traitement des varices par phlébectomie ambulatoire. *Phlébologie* 1966;19:277-9.

In: Varicose Veins   ISBN 978-1-61209-841-8
Editor: Andrea L. Nelson   2011 Nova Science Publishers, Inc.

Chapter 7

THE PATHOGENESIS OF VARICOSE VEINS: "BEYOND VALVULAR INSUFFICIENCY"

*Joseph J. Naoum[1] and Glenn C. Hunter[*2]*

[1]Weill-Cornell Medical College, The Methodist Hospital, Division of
Vascular Surgery, Cardiovascular Surgery Associates, Houston, Texas
[2]Southern Arizona VA Healthcare System and University of Arizona,
Tucson, Arizona, USA

ABSTRACT

Varicose veins (VVs) are commonly attributed to valvular
incompetence resulting in reflux and retrograde venous dilatation. The
occurrence of VVs in the absence of sapheno-femoral (SF), sapheno–
popliteal (SP) or perforator incompetence (IC), and alterations in the
collagen and elastin content of the extracellular matrix (ECM) has lead
investigators to postulate that other, as yet poorly defined local and
systemic factors may act individually or in concert to alter the structural
integrity and function of the venous wall. The clinical and histological
manifestations of VVs occur as a result of the disruption of the normal
venous architecture due to remodeling of the ECM. Persistence of these
systemic and local factors may predispose to the high rates of residual
and recurrent varicosities seen after treatment. Although a number of
growth factors, proteases and their inhibitors known to modulate the

* Correspondence: Glenn C Hunter, MD, 3601 S 6th Ave., Tucson, Arizona 85723, Phone 520-
792-1450 x 6596, Fax 520-629-4603, Cell 520-300-1246

ECM have been implicated in the pathogenesis of VVs, their etiology remains unknown. The identification of potential candidate genes and specific cell markers expressed in response physiologic or pharmacologic stimuli and hemodynamic forces may provide additional insights into the factors that regulate remodeling of the ECM` and ultimately to the development of VVs.

Keywords: varicose veins, prevalence, pathogenesis, matrix remodeling, MMPs, growth factors, venous remodeling

INTRODUCTION

Varicose veins (VVs), an early manifestation of chronic venous disease (CVD) are an important cause of morbidity and escalating health care costs in industrialized western nations. It is estimated that the treatment of patients with CVD accounts for ~2 to 2.6% of the annual health care budget of the United States, France and the United Kingdom (1-3).

DEFINITION AND PATHOGENESIS

CVD is classified according to: clinical signs and symptoms, etiology, anatomic distribution and the pathologic dysfunction (CEAP grades 0-6). The clinical spectrum of CVD ranges from Class (C) $_{0-1}$ no evidence of venous disease; or telangiectasias and reticular veins; C $_{2,3}$ VVs with mild edema to C $_{4,5,6}$ manifest by pigmentation, lipodermatosclerosis and ulceration. The venous abnormalities of CVD range from: telangiectasias "dilated intradermal venules" <1 mm in diameter, reticular veins "dilated and non-palpable subdermal veins 1-3 mm in diameter and", VVs defined as "dilated palpable veins >3 mm in diameter", The term chronic venous insufficiency (CVI) implies a functional abnormality of the venous system and is reserved for advanced disease characterized by edema (C_3), skin changes (C_4) or ulceration ($C_{5,6}$) (4).

PREVALENCE

The prevalence of CVI ranges from <1%-40% in females and <1%-17% in males (5-8). The majority of the patients with CVI (83.4%) are in grades C_3-C_6: (62.8% in grade 3 and 16.3% in grade 4) (9). The prevalence of VVs ranges from 0.1-60.5% in women to 56% in men (10).

The risk factors for VVs are listed in Table 1. Carpentier et al. (11) found that a history of VVs in first degree relatives and age were among the two most important risk factors for developing VVs in either sex (10, 12). Forty-two percent of Japanese patients with VVs have a positive family history compared to 14% of individuals without a family history of varicosities (13). The prevalence of VVs increases from 11.5% in individuals aged 18-24 years to 55.7% in those 55-64 years of age (1). In the United States, the prevalence VVs ranges from <1% in men and 10% in women <30 years of age compared with 57% and 77% in men and women over 70 years of age, respectively (14). The severity of VVs increases with successive pregnancies.

Table 1. Risk Factors for Varicose Veins

Common	Unusual
Genetic predisposition	Connective tissue disorders
Age	Klippel -Trenaunay syndrome, FOXC2 mutation
Female gender	Chuvash polycythemia, NOTCH3 mutation
Multiparity	Vulvo- perineal varicosities
Body mass index	Interosseous perforator vein (IC)
Sedentary occupation	Porto-systemic and Right-Left shunts
Deep venous disease	Persistant sciatic vein (IC)

Contributory factors include; the elevation in intra-abdominal pressure; expansion in blood volume and the increase in venous capacitance and relaxation in response to hemodynamic and hormonal changes accompanying pregnancy (15, 16). Individuals with a body mass index (BMI) of >25 have a higher incidence of CVD, which resolves in most patients after bariatric surgery (17, 18). The calf muscle pump is the major determinant of venous return in the lower extremities. Venous hypertension results in structural changes in the gastrocnemius muscles of patients with CVI and may aggravate the sequelae of valvular incompetence and increase the severity of symptoms associated with prolonged sitting or reduced standing (8, 19). Symptoms can be improved by a structured exercise program that enhances dynamic calf muscle strength and pump function (20). The natural adaptation of the squatting position during defecation and parturition may in part explain the lower incidence of VVs among African nations compared to their Western counterparts.

PATHOPHYSIOLOGY

The superficial and deep veins of the lower extremity communicate via communicating or perforating veins. The direction of flow is normally from the superficial to the deep system aided by the presence of valves and the function of the calf muscle pump. Valvular dysfunction due to their congenital absence, scarring or atrophy, deep venous obstruction or ineffective function of the calf muscle pump results in venous hypertension and if prolonged, attenuation and dilatation of the venous wall (21-24). VVs in younger patients involve the long (LSV), and short (SSV) saphenous veins or their tributaries and maybe either primary (79%) or secondary (post thrombotic 18 %). Older individuals are more likely to have involvement of both LSV and SSV and their tributaries (25-28). In recent reviews of the patterns of reflux in patients with VVs Labropoulos et al. (28) and Engelhorn et al. (25) found that in the majority of patients the disease was distal and segmental with LSV junction involved in <5% of patients. Clinical observations and imaging and histologic studies have challenged the validity of the sapheno-centric theory of VVs popularized by Trendelenberg. He postulated that valvular incompetence and venous dilatation was due to reflux at the sapheno-femoral (SFJ) or sapheno-popliteal junctions (SPJ) and if prolonged, resulted in further separation of the valve cusps, worsening incompetence distally and retrograde progression of CVD (29).

Evidence supporting an increase in hydrostatic pressure and a defect in the structural components of the media as the primary underlying cause of VVs includes: the occurrence of SV in-competence in the absence of reflux at the SFJ in 26.6-67% or SPJ in 42% of patients; the observation that varicosities often precede valvular incompetence and occur below competent valves. Venous dilatation is often observed distal to rather than proximal to a valve, which one would expect if valvular dysfunction was the initiating event. The LSV is normal in 44% of limbs and isolated tributary IC is present in 61% of limbs especially in younger subjects (Figure 1). Superficial venous tributaries behind the knee, lower thigh and upper calf emerging from the subcutaneous tissue of the popliteal fossa, unrelated to the SSV were found in 20% of 444 operative procedures reported by Dodd (26). The exact role of venous hypertension in the development of VV remains unclear since the largest varicosities affecting the lower extremities are not always located in the most dependent segments of the leg exposed to the highest pressures.

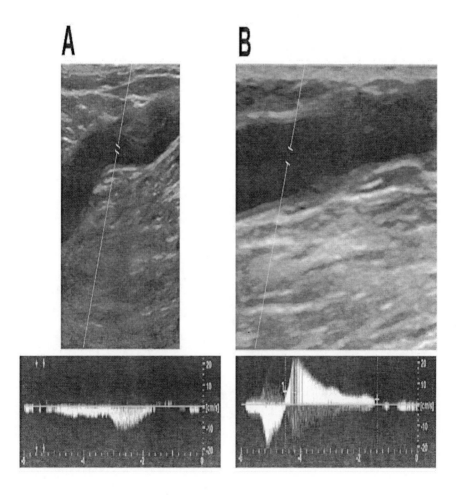

Figure 1. Duplex ultrasound of a varicose long saphenous vein showing a competent segment (A) above an area of reflux (B).

The high venous hydrostatic pressure in the distal parts of the leg results in venous dilation, valvular incompetence, and reflux resulting in reversed flow in below knee perforators and antegrade progression of VVs (Figure 2). Labropoulos, in a study of 116 limbs, examined twice over a 19-month interval found proximal progression of VVs due to new sites of reflux (14 limbs) and reflux progression (17 limbs) in patients awaiting surgery (30-34).

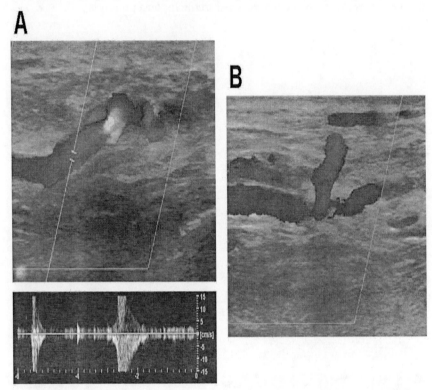

Figure 2. A color flow duplex scan demonstrates (A) a mildly incompetent posterior tibial vein and (B) venous perforator.

The attenuation of the medial layers of the venous wall in patients with VVs is thought to result from the interaction of multiple etiological factors including: the over-expression of genes regulating of the composition of the ECM, increased venous hydrostatic pressure inducing neutrophil and monocyte sequestration and activation, defects in collagen and elastin synthesis and degradation and an imbalance between tissue inhibitors of metalloproteinases (TIMPs) and matrix metalloproteinases (MMPs) in favor of matrix accumulation.

GENETIC ASSOCIATIONS IN VVS

Studies comparing gene expression in VVs and normal SV have shown differential expression of several candidate genes including: actin, transforming growth factor β induced gene, tubulin, desmuslin, versican, type 1 collagen, tenacin, tropomyosin, that regulate SMC function, the assembly of contractile proteins and mineralization [matrix Gla protein (MGP)] in the venous wall (35-40). Tropomyosin 4 regulates the assembly of the contractile mechanisms in the venous wall. The FOXC2 gene, located on chromosome 16q24 encodes a regulatory transcription factor commonly found in patients with lymphedema-distichiasis (VVs in 50%), that plays a role in the development of valves in the venous and lymphatic systems. Notch 3 in patients with cerebral autosomal dominant arteriopathy and the 1208/1209 TT deletion on the thrombomodulin gene have both been associated with the degeneration of SMCs and attenuation of the venous wall in VVs (36, 41). VVs exhibit transcriptional elevation of vascular endothelial growth factor (VEGF)-$_{121,165}$, and its receptors VEGFR-1 and VEGFR-2. In the presence of normal valve function, the transcription of VEGFR-1 remains unaltered. Neuropilin 1 (NRP-1) functions as an isoform-specific receptor for VEGF-$_{165}$ in ECs and as a co-receptor of VEGFR-2 *in vitro* (42, 43). The differential expression of VEGF and its receptors and their interaction with Neuropilin-1 may play a role in the adaptive response of the vein to different stimuli.

HISTOLOGY

Normal SV is composed of intimal, medial and adventitial layers. The intima consists of a lining of ECs overlying a basement membrane and internal elastic lamina. The media is comprised of 3 layers of smooth muscle arranged in bundles: an inner longitudinal layer thickened at valve sites, a well-developed circular middle layer and outer longitudinal layer. The inner and outer muscle layers interdigitate with scaffolds of ECM composed of collagen, elastin, SMCs, fibronectin and proteoglycans. The adventitia is composed of irregular longitudinal muscle fibers, collagen, fibroblasts, SMCs and vasa vasorum. Histologically, VVs are characterized by disruption of the normal venous architecture with areas of intimal thickening (IT) interspersed with normal appearing intima. Desquamation of the endothelial surface with thrombus in various stages of organization is not an infrequent finding (44).

The most prominent histologic feature of VVs is an increase in collagen I in the media. Medial SMCs appear enlarged and display an intermediate state between their proliferative synthetic and contractile phenotypes (45-50). Xiao et al (51) using SMCs isolated from VVs demonstrated a significant increase in proliferative activity [2-fold]; SMC migration and MMP-2 production [3-fold] and collagen synthesis [>2-fold] and decreased expression of phenotypic dependent markers; α smooth muscle actin [α,SM actin] smooth muscle myosin heavy chain [SM-MHC] and smoothelin compared with SMCs derived from normal vein. Treatment of normal SV cells with desmuslin siRNA resulted in a significant increase in collagen synthesis and MMP-2 levels, and a decrease in phenotypic SMC expression characteristic of VVs in culture (52). These data suggest that desmuslin is required for maintenance of SMC phenotype. SMCs and fibroblasts from patients with VVs produce significantly greater amounts of collagen 1 than collagen III and fibronectin, than controls. The increase in collagen I contribute to the separation and disruption of SMC bundles in the media (53, 54). The changes in collagen type 1 and type 111 occur despite comparable levels of mRNAs suggesting a dysregulation of posttranslational synthesis or degradation of these matrix protein components (53, 54). Alterations in the collagen I/III ratio may also contribute to the distensibility and decreased elasticity of the venous wall in VVs. Elastin is increased in the initial phases of the development of VVs and confined to the internal and external lamellae (55). Fragmentation of the elastic lamellae and a reduction in expression of elastin and its precursors occurs with disease progression and increasing age, further contributing to attenuation and dilation of the venous wall (Figure 3) (49, 56). The adventitia of VVs is characterized by an increase in SMCs, fibroblasts, and connective tissue with regions of atrophy and a paucity of vasa vasora. Transmission electron microscopy of VVs shows separation of SMC bundles in the media within a matrix of disorganized collagen fibers. Areas of thinning or blow-out are devoid of SMC and are comprised mostly of collagen fibers lined by a thickened intima and an atrophic adventitia devoid of vasa vasorum (48, 57). Whether the decrease in SMC number, the loss of the connection between SMC and elastin fibers, or an increase in elastase activity is responsible for the elastic fiber derangement in VVs is currently under investigation (56, 58).

TGF-β plays an important role in vascular remodeling and is over expressed in tortuous or hypertrophic VV segments compared to normal vein. TGF-β synthesis and activity usually favors fibrogenesis by perturbing the balance between protease/protease inhibitor activity in favor of collagen synthesis. TGF-β has also been shown to upregulate MMPs favoring matrix degradation in other experimental models. The precise role of TGF-β in the initiation and progression of VVs awaits further study (59).

An imbalance in the expression of matrix metalloproteinases (MMPs) and their inhibitors TIMP-1 and TIMP-2 has been documented in several analyses of VVs (43, 53, 54, 60-64). The expression of MMP-1, MMP-3 and MMP-13 in ECs, medial SMCs, fibroblasts and rare adventitial microvessels is significantly increased in VVs (60).Tissue levels of pro-MMP-2 are increased in the absence of significant changes in MMP-2 expression or activity (54, 62). Plasma levels of pro-MMP-9 and l-Selectin are significantly increased in blood samples obtained from VVs patients after 30 minutes sitting or standing compared to brachial vein samples and MMP-9 protein expression is variable and not significantly changed in VVs (59). Recently, Rafetto et al (65) demonstrated a correlation between the over expression of MMP 2 and MMP 9 and venous wall tension. The authors observed that the MMP 2, induced by an increase in wall tension was associated with venous relaxation and postulate that venous hypertension may induce changes in the ECM by the increase in MMP 2 production. MMP-12 expression is similar to normal veins and localizes to SMCs and fibroblasts (65). TIMPs regulate and maintain the extracellular matrix expression of MMP-1,-2,-9,-12 (64, 66). The expression of TIMP-1 is increased and the quantity and activity of MMP-2 decreased in VVS compared to control vein; whereas, TIMP-2 expression remained unaltered (66). Recently, Aravind et al. (67) have reported higher levels of TIMP-2 in the medial layers of VVs compared to veins harvested from the arm or neck. The expression of TIMP-2 and TIMP-3 was higher in hypertrophic than atrophic VV segments. It should be emphasized, however, that reports in the literature of alterations in collagen and elastin content, protease activity and ECM modulation in VVs have produced conflicting results. The reasons for the marked variability in the clinical, biochemical and molecular findings in patients with VVs reported in the literature are partly due to the failure to accurately locate and describe the patterns and extent of venous reflux. The location of venous tissue sampling is often omitted making comparisons between studies difficult. Delineating the cause and location of venous valvular incompetence assumes increasing importance if the high incidence of residual or recurrent varicosities is to be reduced.

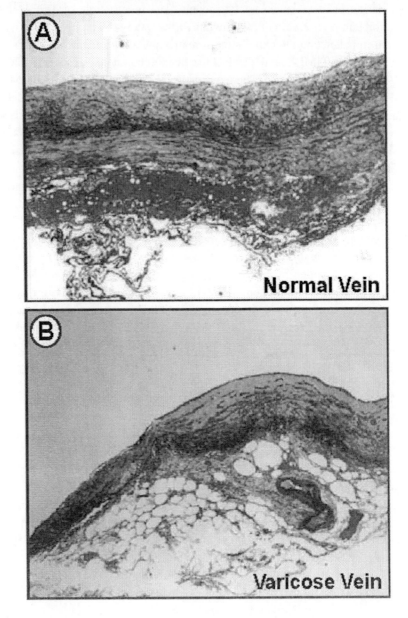

Figure 3. Histological section of a normal (A) and varicose (B) saphenous vein demonstrating loss of the normal venous architecture and attenuation of the wall in the VV section. (Verhoeffs-Van Gieson x 40).

CLINICAL PRESENTATION

The symptoms of VVs result from reflux, obstruction or a combination of both in either the superficial or deep venous systems. McLafferty et al. (68), in a pilot screening study of 476 patients for CVD, found VVs in 32%, edema without skin changes in 11%, skin changes associated with venous disease in 8% and healed or active venous ulceration in 1.3%. The majority of individuals with VVs suffer no medical harm from their varicosities throughout their lifetime. Concerns about the cosmetic appearance, the perceived potential of thrombo-embolic complications, aching or heaviness of the extremity, superficial thrombophlebitis, bleeding, lipodermatosclerosis and ulceration are among the reasons patients seek medical consultation.

DIAGNOSTIC ASSESSMENT

The tortuosity, elongation and dilatation characteristic of VVs usually involve the long and short saphenous veins and their tributaries (25, 31, 69). Sacculation and eventually aneurysmal formation may occur at the SFJ and SPJ or along the course of the SV in the thigh if present for a long time. Careful identification of the sites of valvular incompetence is of fundamental importance in the evaluation and treatment of patients with VVs. Color flow duplex imaging is the gold standard and should be performed in all patients being considered for treatment of their VVs. Patients with VVs should be examined in the standing position with transducer frequencies between 5 and 10 MHZ to detect deep and superficial reflux. The duration of reversed flow should be measured with a pulsed Doppler with either manual or cuff compression and release. The cutoff value for reflux in superficial veins is > 0.5 sec, deep femoral veins > 1.0 sec and >0.35 sec for outward flow in the perforating veins (70). Phlebography is only rarely necessary in patients with complex problems who have associated deep venous disease. Recently CT Phlebography with 3D reconstruction has been used for planning therapeutic interventions (12, 71).

MANAGEMENT OF VVs

An awareness of the anatomical variations in the distribution of varicosities is important when planning treatment for patients with VVs. The indications for treatment of VVs are pain, fatigability, heaviness, recurrent superficial thrombophlebitis, bleeding and ulceration with superficial reflux and cosmetic appearance. The treatment objectives in the management of patients with VVs include: 1) *treatment of the valvular incompetence, and* 2) *obliteration of the venous tributaries*. In essence, the goal of treatment is to redirect flow from the superficial to the deep system. Only a brief outline of the various modalities available to treat VVs will be discussed. Treatment options include: conservative treatment-reassurance and compression therapy; conventional and foam sclerotherapy; ligation of the SFJ and its groin tributaries in conjunction with stab avulsions; endovenous radiofrequency or laser ablation and alternative therapies.

CONSERVATIVE TREATMENT

Conservative management of VVs includes a discussion of the causes and complications of CVD, the benefits of elevation and exercise and elastic support hose and reassurance that complications and progression can be controlled. Patients with a family history of VVs are often concerned that they will develop ulceration or some other complication observed in family members. Allaying such fears and reassurance may be all that is required in some patients. Exercise programs to increase the efficacy of the calf muscle pump can improve the symptoms associated with CVI. Elastic compression stockings or compression therapy narrows the veins, decreases venous volume, and reduces venous reflux by shifting blood volume from the compressed distal extremity centrally. There is also some evidence that compression therapy may also improve calf muscle pump function (72). Although compression therapy alone or in combination with other therapies is effective in reducing swelling and relieving pain, physician advice and patient compliance with elevation and exercise is usually sporadic and evidence of efficacy is often lacking.

SCLEROTHERAPY

Reticular veins, telangiectasias, or "spider" veins respond well to sclerotherapy. The smaller the vein, the better the response to treatment. Sclerotherapy can relieve pain and prevent ulceration and venous hemorrhage (73-75). Compression sclerotherapy has also been used to obliterate VVs in the outpatient setting. The popularity of sclerotherapy has declined over the years because of poor long-term efficacy and increased incidence of superficial thrombophlebitis and thrombo-embolism associated with the volume of sclerosant used to obliterate large varicosities below the knee. In a comparison of sclerotherapy with support hose, Abramovitz et al. (76) showed an advantage for empty vein compressive sclerotherapy in the relief of symptoms and improved cosmetic appearance in pregnant women. A Cochrane review of the efficacy of sclerotherapy in the treatment of VVs found only limited benefit and the results of poor quality (77). A number of studies have compared surgery versus sclerotherapy. Although the overall quality of these studies is somewhat variable, there is a trend toward better results with surgery after 3 years and with significantly lower recurrence rates beyond 5 years. Foam sclerosants can be used in the treatment of small, moderate VVs as well as in the obliteration of larger veins in combination with SFJ ligation (78, 79). In a follow-up study at 5 years Cabrera reported 81% complete fibrosis of the LSV and disappearance of 96% of tributaries (79, 80).

MANAGEMENT OF SAPHENO- FEMORAL INCOMPETENCE

Surgery

The aims of surgical treatment of VVs are: *(1) to obliterate the saphenous vein and (2) remove cluster varicosities*. In a randomized controlled trial (REATIV) evaluating the cost effectiveness of the various treatment modalities for VVs, 79.2% of the patients were found to have reflux in the long saphenous vein (LSV), 68.8% in the groin and LSV above the knee, 21% at the groin only, 10.1% LSV only above the knee and 17.8% had reflux in the popliteal fossa. High ligation of the SFJ, stripping of the SV and stab avulsion of the tributaries is considered the definitive treatment for VVs. The results of surgery are more durable than sclerotherapy, but do involve an inpatient/outpatient procedure. The complication rate for patients undergoing surgery was 12.2% of which wound infection was the most common. The recurrence rate of surgically treated VVs ranges from 20%-80% at 5 and 20 years, respectively. Varicose vein tributaries can be removed by either stab avulsion phlebectomy or with transilluminated power phlebectomy. The latter, also known as TriVex removes clusters of varicosities with fewer incisions and a potential reduction in operating time (74, 75).

RADIO-FREQUENCY AND LASER CLOSURE

Recently minimally invasive outpatient treatment for VVs as an alternative to surgical stripping has been introduced. Radio-frequency or laser ablation using thermal energy is performed under tumescent local anesthesia in the outpatient setting and is effective in obliterating the LSV in the short term. Failure to ablate the saphenous vein and recannalization and persistent reflux occurred in13% and 16% undergoing radiofrequency ablation at 5 years and in 7% of extremities treated with endovenous laser at 2 years (81). Both radio-frequency and Laser closer treatment requires adjunctive treatment of tributary varicosities. Randomized clinical trials comparing these newer forms of treatment versus surgery are essential to determine their long-term durability and cost effectiveness before they can replace surgical treatment.

SAPHENO-POPLITEAL INCOMPETENCE

Incompetence of the SSV has been associated with the manifestations of the entire spectrum of CVD. Reflux in the SSV can be isolated or occur in conjunction with reflux in the LSV in patient with VVs. The treatment of SSV is quite varied due to the lack of definitive clinical trials. A questionnaire survey of the surgical members of the Vascular Surgical Society of Great Britain and Ireland found that only 10.4% of surgeons formally exposed and identified the popliteal vein during SP ligation, the majority (75.7%) dissected down the short saphenous vein to visualize the junction. The short saphenous vein was stripped routinely by 14.5% of surgeons, the majority preferring to excise a proximal segment of up to 10 cm (55.1%) (82).

In a more recent survey, O'hare et al. (83) found that SPJ ligation or SSV stripping was the preferred surgical option in recent prospective UK study. Stripping of the SSV was associated with a reduced rate of SPJ IC at 1 year.

The variation in management of short saphenous veins may be explained by the lack of definitive clinical trials in this area.

ALTERNATIVE THERAPY FOR VVS

Although there have been attempts to link the fiber content of diets to the occurrence of VVs, the association remains rather tenacious. The role of other factors contributing to the occurrence of VVs including cigarette smoking, the use of oral contraceptives, hypertension, and diabetes remains to be validated (6, 10). Thus, behavioral changes targeted at a healthier lifestyle may potentially reduce the incidence of VVs.

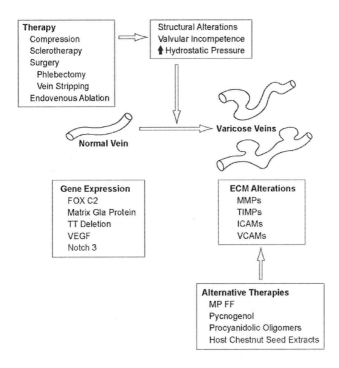

Figure 4. Schematic diagram of the pathologic alterations that lead to venous insufficiency and varicose vein formation as targets for therapeutic intervention. ECM -extracellular matrix, ICAM –intracellular adhesion molecule, MMPs -matrix metalloproteinases, MPFF–micronized purified flavanoid fraction. TIMP-tissue inhibitor of metalloproteinases, VCAM -vascular cell adhesion molecule, VEGF-vascular endothelial growth factor.

The endothelial layer of VVs is characterized by areas of desquamation and degenerative changes in individual ECs under EM. These abnormal ECs, once activated release inflammatory mediators that attract and activate neutrophils resulting in upregulation of the expression of vascular cell adhesion molecule 1(VCAM-1), intracellular adhesion molecule 1ICAM-1) and von Willebrand factor. Activated leucocytes also release free radicals and proteases that degrade the ECM (46). Venous hypertension results in stasis in the microcirculation, reduces shear stress on the ECs and a decrease in cellular levels of NO, a key factor in upregulating adhesion molecule expression and neutrophil activation (84, 85). In addition, activated endothelial cells release growth factors that induce smooth muscle cell migration, proliferation and de-differentiation into the synthetic phenotype, leading to the formation of neointima (46). A number of the alternative therapies have been shown to reduce the inflammatory response induced by venous hypertension and result in symptom relief in patients with VVs (Figure 4). Micronized purified flavanoid fraction (MPFF) and pycnogenol have been demonstrated to reduce the expression of ICAM-1 andVCAM-1 in patients with CVD. MPFF consists of diosmin and flavanoids in the form of hesperidin extracted from *Sophora Japonica*. Mesoglycan, a sulphated polysaccharide, inhibits neutrophil adhesion and results in symptomatic relief in patients with CVD. The maritime pine bark (*Pinus maritime)* extract, pycnogenol has been shown to inhibit the lipoxygenase and prostaglandin pathways. Two metabolites are derived from the oral ingestion of pycnogenol namely delta-(3,4dihydroxyphenyl)-gamma-valerolactone and delta-(3-Methoxy-4-hydroxyphenyl)-gamma-valerolactone. The first has superoxide scavenger activities and both metabolites have shown strong inhibitory effects on MMP1, 2, and 9. These compounds have the potential of serving as protective agents that can influence the activation the inflammatory molecules and cells. They also demonstrate the ability to decrease extremity edema, shorten the time to ulcer healing, and decrease scar formation (86, 87). Phlebotonic drugs such as flavanoids and horse chestnut seed extracts from *Aesculus hippocastanum* contain aescin and flavanoids. The former has been demonstrated to have potent anti-inflammatory activity by closing vascular gaps, decreasing capillary filtration rates, and clinically reducing edema (88). Procyanidolic oligomers support fibroblast synthesis of hyaluronan, proteoglycans, and other matrix proteins in vitro. It can reduce symptoms and edema in patients with CVI (89).

Summary

VVs are the clinical manifestation of valvular insufficiency in the superficial and deep venous system. Female gender, increasing age and a family history are the most frequently associated risk factors. The complex anatomical patterns of venous reflux, changes in hydrostatic pressure, derangements in SMC architecture, and alterations in the ECM and its components are among the etiological factors implicated in the pathogenesis of VVs. The clinical assessment, diagnostic evaluation and treatment of each patient should be individualized to ensure the appropriate treatment with the lowest rate of residual tributaries and recurrence. Although results of the newer methods of saphenous vein ablation at 1 and 5 years are at least good as surgical treatment, controversy remains regarding their cost and durability. Further studies are necessary to elucidate the influence of the hemodynamic derangements on the ECM in the venous wall Delineating the cellular mechanisms resulting in the characteristic features of VVs is imperative in order to develop effective preventive and therapeutic strategies for VVs.

References

[1]   Ruckley CV, Evans CJ, Allan PL, et al. Chronic venous insufficiency: clinical and duplex correlations. The Edinburgh Vein Study of venous disorders in the general population. *J Vasc Surg* 2002; 36:520-525.

[2]   Van den Oever R, Hepp B, Debbaut B, et al. Socio-economic impact of chronic venous insufficiency. An underestimated public health problem. *Int Angiol* 1998; 17:161-167.

[3]   Weingarten MS. State-of-the-art treatment of chronic venous disease. *Clin Infect Dis* 2001; 32:949-954.

[4]   Eklof B, Rutherford RB, Bergan JJ, et al. Revision of the CEAP classification for chronic venous disorders: consensus statement. *J Vasc Surg* 2004; 40:1248-1252.

[5]   Rabe KF, Pannier-Fischer F, Bromen K. Venenstudie der Gesellschaft Fu"r Phlebologie. *Phlebologie* 2003; 32:1-14.

[6]   6Beebe-Dimmer JL, Pfeifer JR, Engle JS, et al. The epidemiology of chronic venous insufficiency and varicose veins. *Ann Epidemiol* 2005; 15:175-184.

[7]   Carpentier PH, Maricq HR, Biro C, et al. Prevalence, risk factors, and clinical patterns of chronic venous disorders of lower limbs: a population-based study in France. *J Vasc Surg* 2004; 40:650-659.

[8]   Evans CJ, Fowkes FG, Ruckley CV, et al. Prevalence of varicose veins and chronic venous insufficiency in men and women in the general population: Edinburgh Vein Study. *J Epidemiol Community Health* 1999; 53:149-153.

[9]   Fiebig A, Krusche P, Wolf A, et al. Heritability of chronic venous disease. *Hum Genet* 2010; 127:669-674.

[10] Robertson L, Evans C, Fowkes FG. Epidemiology of chronic venous disease. *Phlebology* 2008; 23:103-111.

[11] Carpentier PH. [Epidemiology and physiopathology of chronic venous leg diseases]. *Rev Prat* 2000; 50:1176-1181.

[12] Jung SC, Lee W, Chung JW, et al. Unusual causes of varicose veins in the lower extremities: CT venographic and Doppler US findings. *Radiographics* 2009; 29:525-536.

[13] Hirai M, Naiki K, Nakayama R. Prevalence and risk factors of varicose veins in Japanese women. *Angiology* 1990; 41:228-232.

[14] Brand FN, Dannenberg AL, Abbott RD, et al. The epidemiology of varicose veins: the Framingham Study. *Am J Prev Med* 1988; 4:96-101.

[15] Laurikka JO, Sisto T, Tarkka MR, et al. Risk indicators for varicose veins in forty- to sixty-year-olds in the Tampere varicose vein study. *World J Surg* 2002; 26:648-651.

[16] Naoum JJ, Hunter GC, Woodside KJ, et al. Current advances in the pathogenesis of varicose veins. *J Surg Res* 2007; 141:311-316.

[17] Poirier P, Giles TD, Bray GA, et al. Obesity and cardiovascular disease: pathophysiology, evaluation, and effect of weight loss. *Arterioscler Thromb Vasc Biol* 2006; 26:968-976.

[18] Sugerman HJ, Sugerman EL, Wolfe L, et al. Risks and benefits of gastric bypass in morbidly obese patients with severe venous stasis disease. *Ann Surg* 2001; 234:41-46.

[19] Eifell RK, Ashour HY, Heslop PS, et al. Association of 24-hour activity levels with the clinical severity of chronic venous disease. *J Vasc Surg* 2006; 44:580-587.

[20] Padberg FT, Jr., Johnston MV, Sisto SA. Structured exercise improves calf muscle pump function in chronic venous insufficiency: a randomized trial. *J Vasc Surg* 2004; 39:79-87.

[21] Ascher E, Jacob T, Hingorani A, et al. Expression of molecular mediators of apoptosis and their role in the pathogenesis of lower-extremity varicose veins. *J Vasc Surg* 2001; 33:1080-1086.

[22] Blanchemaison P. [Significance of venous endoscopy in the exploration and the treatment of venous insufficiency of the legs]. *J Mal Vasc* 1992; 17 Suppl B:109-112.

[23] Corcos L, De Anna D, Dini M, et al. Proximal long saphenous vein valves in primary venous insufficiency. *J Mal Vasc* 2000; 25:27-36.

[24] Van Cleef JF, Hugentobler JP, Desvaux P, et al. [Endoscopic study of reflux of the saphenous valve]. *J Mal Vasc* 1992; 17 Suppl B:113-116.

[25] Engelhorn CA, Engelhorn AL, Cassou MF, et al. Patterns of saphenous reflux in women with primary varicose veins. *J Vasc Surg* 2005; 41:645-651.

[26] Dodd H. The varicose tributaries of the popliteal vein. *Br J Surg* 1965; 52:350-354.

[27] Kistner RL, Eklof B, Masuda EM. Diagnosis of chronic venous disease of the lower extremities: the "CEAP" classification. *Mayo Clin Proc* 1996; 71:338-345.

[28] Labropoulos N, Kokkosis AA, Spentzouris G, et al. The distribution and significance of varicosities in the saphenous trunks. *J Vasc Surg* 2010; 51:96-103.

[29] Trendelenberg F. Uber die Tunderbindung der Vena Saphena Magna bie unterschenkel Varicen. *Beitt Z Clin Chir* 1980; 7:195.

[30] Bernardini E, Piccioli R, De Rango P, et al. Echo-sclerosis hemodynamic conservative: a new technique for varicose vein treatment. *Ann Vasc Surg* 2007; 21:535-543.

[31] Caggiati A, Rosi C, Heyn R, et al. Age-related variations of varicose veins anatomy. *J Vasc Surg* 2006; 44:1291-1295.

[32] Labropoulos N, Tassiopoulos AK, Bhatti AF, et al. Development of reflux in the perforator veins in limbs with primary venous disease. *J Vasc Surg* 2006; 43:558-562.

[33] Pittaluga P, Chastanet S, Guex JJ. Great saphenous vein stripping with preservation of sapheno-femoral confluence: hemodynamic and clinical results. *J Vasc Surg* 2008; 47:1300-1304; discussion 1304-1305.

[34] Labropoulos N, Leon L, Kwon S, et al. Study of the venous reflux progression. *J Vasc Surg* 2005; 41:291-295.

[35] Kim DI, Eo HS, Joh JH. Identification of differentially expressed genes in primary varicose veins. *J Surg Res* 2005; 123:222-226.

[36] Lim CS, Davies AH. Pathogenesis of primary varicose veins. *Br J Surg* 2009; 96:1231-1242.

[37] Mellor RH, Brice G, Stanton AW, et al. Mutations in FOXC2 are strongly associated with primary valve failure in veins of the lower limb. *Circulation* 2007; 115:1912-1920.

[38] Ng MY, Andrew T, Spector TD, et al. Linkage to the FOXC2 region of chromosome 16 for varicose veins in otherwise healthy, unselected sibling pairs. *J Med Genet* 2005; 42:235-239.

[39] Yin H, Zhang X, Wang J, et al. Downregulation of desmuslin in primary vein incompetence. *J Vasc Surg* 2006; 43:372-378.

[40] Cario-Toumaniantz C, Boularan C, Schurgers LJ, et al. Identification of differentially expressed genes in human varicose veins: involvement of matrix gla protein in extracellular matrix remodeling. *J Vasc Res* 2007; 44:444-459.

[41] Le Flem L, Mennen L, Aubry ML, et al. Thrombomodulin promoter mutations, venous thrombosis, and varicose veins. *Arterioscler Thromb Vasc Biol* 2001; 21:445-451.

[42] Hollingsworth SJ, Powell G, Barker SG, et al. Primary varicose veins: altered transcription of VEGF and its receptors (KDR, flt-1, soluble flt-1) with sapheno-femoral junction incompetence. *Eur J Vasc Endovasc Surg* 2004; 27:259-268.

[43] Woodside KJ, Naoum JJ, Torry RJ, et al. Altered expression of vascular endothelial growth factor and its receptors in normal saphenous vein and in arterialized and stenotic vein grafts. *Am J Surg* 2003; 186:561-568.

[44] Wali MA, Dewan M, Eid RA. Histopathological changes in the wall of varicose veins. *Int Angiol* 2003; 22:188-193.

[45] London NJ, Nash R. ABC of arterial and venous disease. Varicose veins. *BMJ* 2000; 320:1391-1394.

[46] Michiels C, Bouaziz N, Remacle J. Role of the endothelium and blood stasis in the development of varicose veins. *Int Angiol* 2002; 21:18-25.

[47] Milroy CM, Scott DJ, Beard JD, et al. Histological appearances of the long saphenous vein. *J Pathol* 1989; 159:311-316.

[48] Rose SS, Ahmed A. Some thoughts on the aetiology of varicose veins. *J Cardiovasc Surg (Torino)* 1986; 27:534-543.

[49] Venturi M, Bonavina L, Annoni F, et al. Biochemical assay of collagen and elastin in the normal and varicose vein wall. *J Surg Res* 1996; 60:245-248.

[50] Moneta GL, Hehler M. The lower extremity venous system: Anatomy and physiology of normal venous function and chronic venous insufficiency. In: Handbook of Venous Disorders. London: Chapman & Hall; 1986.

[51] Xiao Y, Huang Z, Yin H, et al. In vitro differences between smooth muscle cells derived from varicose veins and normal veins. *J Vasc Surg* 2009; 50:1149-1154.

[52] Xiao Y, Huang Z, Yin H, et al. Desmuslin gene knockdown causes altered expression of phenotype markers and differentiation of saphenous vein smooth muscle cells. *J Vasc Surg* 2010; 52:684-690.

[53] Sansilvestri-Morel P, Nonotte I, Fournet-Bourguignon MP, et al. Abnormal deposition of extracellular matrix proteins by cultured smooth muscle cells from human varicose veins. *J Vasc Res* 1998; 35:115-123.

[54] Sansilvestri-Morel P, Rupin A, Jaisson S, et al. Synthesis of collagen is dysregulated in cultured fibroblasts derived from skin of subjects with varicose veins as it is in venous smooth muscle cells. *Circulation* 2002; 106:479-483.

[55] Kirsch D, Schreiber J, Dienes HP, et al. Alterations of the extracellular matrix of venous walls in varicous veins. *Vasa* 1999; 28:95-99.

[56] Bujan J, Gimeno MJ, Jimenez JA, et al. Expression of elastic components in healthy and varicose veins. *World J Surg* 2003; 27:901-905.

[57] Elsharawy MA, Naim MM, Abdelmaguid EM, et al. Role of saphenous vein wall in the pathogenesis of primary varicose veins. *Interact Cardiovasc Thorac Surg* 2007; 6:219-224.

[58] Kockx MM, Knaapen MW, Bortier HE, et al. Vascular remodeling in varicose veins. *Angiology* 1998; 49:871-877.

[59] Jacob MP, Cazaubon M, Scemama A, et al. Plasma matrix metalloproteinase-9 as a marker of blood stasis in varicose veins. *Circulation* 2002; 106:535-538.

[60] Gillespie DL, Patel A, Fileta B, et al. Varicose veins possess greater quantities of MMP-1 than normal veins and demonstrate regional variation in MMP-1 and MMP-13. *J Surg Res* 2002; 106:233-238.

[61] Hanemaaijer R, Koolwijk P, le Clercq L, et al. Regulation of matrix metalloproteinase expression in human vein and microvascular endothelial cells. Effects of tumour necrosis factor alpha, interleukin 1 and phorbol ester. *Biochem J* 1993; 296 (Pt 3):803-809.

[62] Kowalewski R, Sobolewski K, Wolanska M, et al. Matrix metalloproteinases in the vein wall. *Int Angiol* 2004; 23:164-169.

[63] Kosugi I, Urayama H, Kasashima F, et al. Matrix metalloproteinase-9 and urokinase-type plasminogen activator in varicose veins. *Ann Vasc Surg* 2003; 17:234-238.

[64] Parra JR, Cambria RA, Hower CD, et al. Tissue inhibitor of metalloproteinase-1 is increased in the saphenofemoral junction of patients with varices in the leg. *J Vasc Surg* 1998; 28:669-675.

[65] Raffetto JD, Qiao X, Koledova VV, et al. Prolonged increases in vein wall tension increase matrix metalloproteinases and decrease constriction in rat vena cava: Potential implications in varicose veins. *J Vasc Surg* 2008; 48:447-456.

[66] Badier-Commander C, Verbeuren T, Lebard C, et al. Increased TIMP/MMP ratio in varicose veins: a possible explanation for extracellular matrix accumulation. *J Pathol* 2000; 192:105-112.

[67] Aravind B, Saunders B, Navin T, et al. Inhibitory effect of TIMP influences the morphology of varicose veins. *Eur J Vasc Endovasc Surg* 2010; 40:754-765.

[68] McLafferty RB, Lohr JM, Caprini JA, et al. Results of the national pilot screening program for venous disease by the American Venous Forum. *J Vasc Surg* 2007; 45:142-148.

[69] Labropoulos N, Leon L, Engelhorn CA, et al. Sapheno-femoral junction reflux in patients with a normal saphenous trunk. *Eur J Vasc Endovasc Surg* 2004; 28:595-599.

[70] Labropoulos N, Tiongson J, Pryor L, et al. Definition of venous reflux in lower-extremity veins. *J Vasc Surg* 2003; 38:793-798.

[71] Min SK, Kim SY, Park YJ, et al. Role of three-dimensional computed tomography venography as a powerful navigator for varicose vein surgery. *J Vasc Surg* 2010; 51:893-899.

[72] Nicolaides AN. Investigation of chronic venous insufficiency: A consensus statement (France, March 5-9, 1997). *Circulation* 2000; 102:E126-163.

[73] Bartholomew JR, King T, Sahgal A, et al. Varicose veins: newer, better treatments available. *Cleve Clin J Med* 2005; 72:312-314, 319-321, 325-318.

[74] Eberhardt RT, Raffetto JD. Chronic venous insufficiency. *Circulation* 2005; 111:2398-2409.

[75] Nitecki S, Kantarovsky A, Portnoy I, et al. The contemporary treatment of varicose veins (strangle, strip, grill or poison). *Isr Med Assoc J* 2006; 8:411-415.

[76] Abramowitz I. The treatment of varicose veins in pregnancy by empty vein compressive sclerotherapy. *S Afr Med J* 1973; 47:607-610.

[77] Tisi PV, Beverley CA. Injection sclerotherapy for varicose veins (Cochrane Review). *Cochrane Database Syst Rev* 2003; 4:1-78.

[78] Stucker M, Kobus S, Altmeyer P, et al. Review of published information on foam sclerotherapy. *Dermatol Surg* 2010; 36 Suppl 2:983-992.

[79] Thomasset SC, Butt Z, Liptrot S, et al. Ultrasound guided foam sclerotherapy: factors associated with outcomes and complications. *Eur J Vasc Endovasc Surg* 2010; 40:389-392.

[80] Cabrera J, Cabrera JJ. Nueva metodo de esclerosis en las varices tronculares. *Patol Vasc* 1995; 4:55-73.

[81] Merchant RF, Pichot O. Long-term outcomes of endovenous radiofrequency obliteration of saphenous reflux as a treatment for superficial venous insufficiency. *J Vasc Surg* 2005; 42:502-509; discussion 509.

[82] Winterborn RJ, Campbell WB, Heather BP, et al. The management of short saphenous varicose veins: a survey of the members of the vascular surgical society of Great Britain and Ireland. *Eur J Vasc Endovasc Surg* 2004; 28:400-403.

[83] O'Hare JL, Vandenbroeck CP, Whitman B, et al. A prospective evaluation of the outcome after small saphenous varicose vein surgery with one-year follow-up. *J Vasc Surg* 2008; 48:669-673; discussion 674.

[84] Grimm T, Schafer A, Hogger P. Antioxidant activity and inhibition of matrix metalloproteinases by metabolites of maritime pine bark extract (pycnogenil). *Free Radic Biol Med* 1999; 27:704-724.

[85] Nikolovska S, Pavlova L, Ancevski A, et al. The role of nitric oxide in the pathogenesis of venous ulcers. *Acta Dermatovenerol Croat* 2005; 13:242-246.

[86] Katsenis K. Micronized purified flavonoid fraction (MPFF): a review of its pharmacological effects, therapeutic efficacy and benefits in the management of chronic venous insufficiency. *Curr Vasc Pharmacol* 2005; 3:1-9.

[87] Wollina U, Abdel-Naser MB, Mani R. A review of the microcirculation in skin in patients with chronic venous insufficiency: the problem and the evidence available for therapeutic options. *Int J Low Extrem Wounds* 2006; 5:169-180.

[88] Sirtori CR. Aescin: pharmacology, pharmacokinetics and therapeutic profile. *Pharmacol Res* 2001; 44:183-193.

[89] Daroczy J, Pal A, Blasko G. Microcirculatory changes in patients with chronic venous and lymphatic insufficiency and heavy leg symptoms before and after therapy with procyanidol oligomers (Laser Doppler study). *Orv Hetil* 2004; 36:811-822.

INDEX

D

E

Q

R

T